Radiation Therapy Essentials
Board Preparation Tool

Anne Marie Vann, MEd., RT (R)(T), CMD
Joan Arazie, BS, RT (R)(T)
Miles Sutton, BS, RT (T)

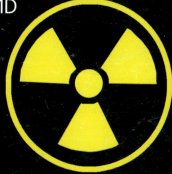

Copyright © 2010 by RadOnc Publications

ISBN: 978-0-615-41665-6
Library of Congress Control Number: 2010940386

All Rights Reserved.
No part of this book may be reproduced in any form or by any means without the prior written consent of RadOnc Publications.

Illustrations by Miles Sutton, BS, RT (T)
Technical Layout by Valene Sims

PREFACE

This book is intended as a refresher for those preparing for board certification or recertification in the field of radiation oncology. Outline format brings key points to the forefront. Examples and diagrams are provided to aid in quick recognition and clarification of the topic.

DISCLAIMER

This textbook does not claim to be all inclusive or void of human error. The authors have made every attempt to confirm the accuracy of the material contained within. There has been no single source used to gather this review material. The reader is encouraged to consult supplemental materials for a deeper investigation of the common facts presented.

The authors realize the normal tissue complication probability is dependent on a variety of factors. We have chosen to list the traditional normal tissue tolerance doses as published by Emami, et. al. (1991) and the National Cancer Institute.

Clinical Concepts in Radiation Oncology

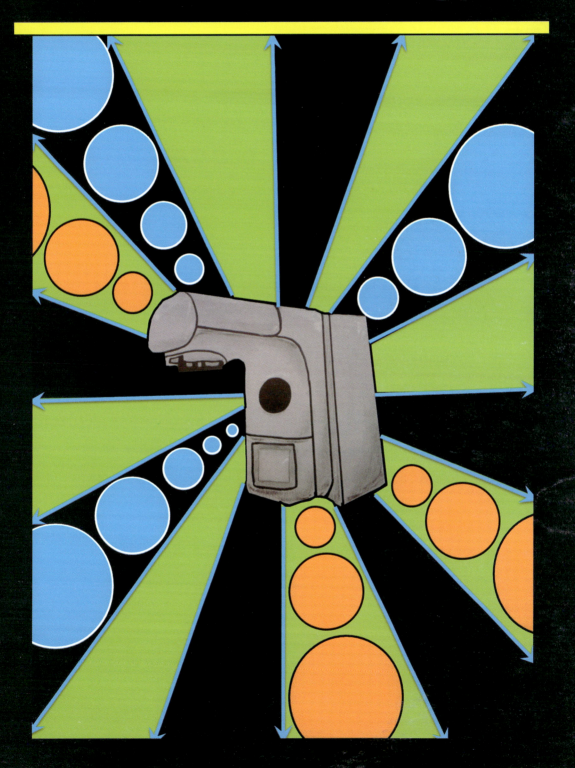

Tumor Classification

- Benign tumors (non-cancerous)
    - Normal to slightly increased growth
    - Encapsulated
    - Well differentiated
    - Not usually life threatening
- Malignant tumors (cancerous)
    - Normal to increased mitotic rate
    - Can metastasize
    - Well differentiated to anaplastic (undifferentiated)
    - Life threatening

Malignant Histopathology

- Carcinomas ($\approx$ 75-85% of tumors)
    - Originate from the epithelium (tissues that cover a surface or line a cavity)
    - Squamous cell carcinomas
    - Glandular cells (adenocarcinomas)
    - Generally spread by lymphatics
- Sarcomas ($\approx$ 10-15% of tumors)
    - Originate from bone, connective, or soft tissue
    - Generally spread through the blood
    - Most common metastatic site is the lungs
- Other Tissue Types ($\approx$ 5-10% of tumors)

Etiology

Study of the cause of disease

- Identifying carcinogens

- Genetic Factors
- Helps to establish screening programs and preventive cancer education

Epidemiology

Study of the incidence of disease

- Factors such as age, gender, race, occupation, and geographic location can determine which type of cancer effects which group of people

Screening Tests

- Prostate – blood PSA (Prostatic Specific Antigen)
- Breast – mammogram
- Cervix – papanicolaou (PAP) smear
- Colorectal Cancer – fecal occult blood, colonoscopy

Cancer Workup

- Biopsy – the ONLY way to definitively diagnose cancer
- Diagnostic tests based on tumor type, location, size, and extent

Diagnostic Tests

- Biopsy – confirm the presence of cancer cells
- X-rays – can be taken of the chest, abdomen, bones, etc. Dye can also be used to better visualize anatomy. X-rays (e.g. barium swallow, IVP, barium enema) can be diagnostic 2D films or performed on a CT scanner to get 3D anatomical information
- Computed Tomography (CT) Scan – x-rays that provide 3D sectional anatomy with good contrast between tissue and bony anatomy
- Magnetic Resonance Imaging (MRI) – uses magnets opposed to radiation to visualize 3D images of anatomy. Provides good contrast between soft tissues
- Visualization/Biopsy through a scope – endoscope, proctoscope, cystoscope
- Nuclear Medicine Studies – uses radioisotopes to visualize anatomy and function. (e.g. PET scan, thyroid scan, bone scan)
- Ultrasound – used for cystic (benign) tumors versus solid (malignant) tumors, and for localization (biopsy, treatment depth)
- Lab Values – tumor markers, kidney, liver, thyroid function, blood values (e.g. WBC, hemoglobin)

Common Staging Systems

The American Joint Committee on Cancer (AJCC) staging is based on size and extent of tumor invasion. The letters T, N, and M are used to stage the tumor

- **T** – Describes the size and invasiveness of the primary tumor. A numerical value (1-4) is added to the T and increases with the extent of the tumor
    - T1 – Small lesion confined to the organ of origin
    - T2 – Larger tumor size or deeper extension
    - T3 – Extension beyond the organ of origin, but confined to the region
    - T4 – Invasion into another organ or viscera
- **N** – Describes the presence or absence of involvement in regional lymph nodes. In some sites, there is an increasing numerical value based on size, fixation, and capsular invasion. In other sites, numerical value is based on multiple node involvement or number of local and regional lymph nodes
- **M** – Describes the presence or absence of distant metastasis, including lymph nodes that are not regional

General staging terms:

- **In-situ** – means "in-place", non-invasive, pre-invasive, or stage 0. Malignant cells still resemble cell group from which they arose. There is no penetration of the basement membrane of the tissue and no stromal invasion. In-situ describes carcinomas or melanomas only (does not describe sarcomas)
- **Localized** – A malignancy limited to the organ of origin, infiltration past the basement membrane of epithelium into the stroma of the organ. The tumor can be widely invasive or even show metastasis within the organ itself and still be considered localized
- **Regionalized** – Tumor extension beyond limits of organ of origin. Includes a portion of, or an entire organ with outer limits to include at least the first level of lymph nodes
- **Distant** – A tumor which has spread to distant areas of the body, distant or remote from the primary tumor. Tumor cells have broken away from the primary tumor and traveled to distant parts of the body, there is normal tissue intervening. Distant is also known as disseminated, diffuse, or metastatic
- **Unknown** – Cancer is staged as unknown or unstageable if sufficient information cannot be obtained. The symbol "X" is used to denote a tumor that is undetermined or unable to assess stage

FIGO Staging for Gynecological (GYN) Tumors

- A system approved by the International Federation of Gynecologists and Obstetricians (FIGO) for staging a particular gynecologic cancer. Uses Roman numerals and numbers to designate the size and extent of the cancer. The staging is based on the clinical examination prior to the definitive treatment for control and cure

Duke Staging of Colorectal Cancer

- Numbers I-IV are used to designate the extent of cancer based on resection of the tumor and the depth of invasion through the mucosa and bowel wall. (The TNM staging system is used more frequently than Duke for colorectal cancers)

Ann Arbor Lymphoma Staging

- The staging system for both Hodgkin Lymphoma and Non-Hodgkin Lymphoma (NHL). Numbers I-IV designates the extent of disease. The letters A and B designate the presence (B) or absence (A) of symptoms. B symptoms include: unexplained weight loss (greater than 10% of body weight), fevers greater than 101°, and drenching night sweats

Melanoma Staging

- Breslow thickness is defined as the total vertical height of the melanoma from the top of the area to the deepest penetration into the skin. The higher the Breslow thickness, the worse the prognosis

- Clark level of invasion is how deep the tumor has penetrated into the layers of the skin. Not as useful as Breslow staging

Grading (not to be confused with staging)

- Based on microscopic appearance

- Shows the degree of differentiation at a cellular level

- Can be a major prognostic indicator

- G0-G4 grading ranges from well differentiated (G0) to Anaplastic (G4) in appearance, and slow growth to high mitotic rate (GX is given when grade is unable to be assessed)

Treatment Options

- Surgery, radiation therapy, chemotherapy, hormone therapy (e.g. prostate and breast), immunotherapy (biotherapy)

Treatment Results

- The Surveillance, Epidemiology, and End Results (SEER) program of the National Cancer Institute (NCI) provides information on cancer incidence and survival in the United States. SEER collects and publishes data from cancer registries in the United States

Head and Neck Cancers

Risk factors

- Smoking is the number one risk factor for head and neck cancers

- Smoking and alcohol can have a *synergistic* effect (the combination of these two risk factors used together can cause a greater chance of cancer)

- More common in men (except thyroid cancer) and the elderly

Most common routes of spread

- Direct invasion and spread by the lymphatics (carcinomas)

- The jugulodigastric nodes (JD nodes) are the most commonly involved lymph nodes. The JD nodes are located at the angle of the mandible

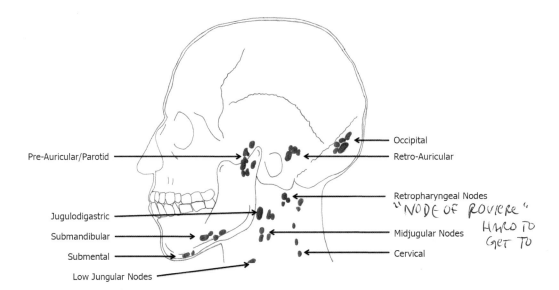

Treatment options

- Surgery, radiation therapy, and chemotherapy are options in all head and neck regions, unless noted

Critical structures and Tolerance Doses

Organ	Tolerance Dose	Endpoint
Spinal Cord	4700 cGy	Necrosis
Lens	1000 cGy	Cataracts
Lacrimal Gland	2600 cGy	Dry Eye
Optic Chiasm	5000 cGy	Blindness
Optic Nerve	5000 cGy	Blindness
Paraotid Gland	3200 cGy	Xerostomia
Temporomandibular Joint	6000 cGy	Limitation of joint function
Esophagus	5500 cGy	Stricture/Perforation
Thyroid	4500 cGy	Thyroiditis
Larynx	4500 cGy	Edema
Ear	3000 / 5500 cGy	Acute/Chronic Serious Otitis

Acute Radiation Reactions

- Mucositis – inflammation of the mucus membrane

- Parotitis – may occur 8-10 hours after radiation. Painful, swollen parotid gland. This is temporary and is usually resolved in a matter of hours

- Laryngeal Edema – edema of the arytenoids

Acute and Chronic Radiation Reactions

- Xerostomia - dryness of the mucous membranes in the oral cavity

- Dental Caries – vascular damage, reduced salvia and poor dental hygiene contribute to dental caries

- Trismus – fibrosis around the masticatory muscles and temporomandibular joint

- Subcutaneous Fibrosis – hardening of the skin

- Endocrine dysfunction – occurs when >75% of endocrine glands are irradiated at high doses

Rare Complications

- Osteoradionecrosis (of the mandible) – occurs with high doses >6000 cGy. Damages the vasculature of the bone and protective covering and the bone cannot resist trauma or infection

- Soft Tissue Necrosis

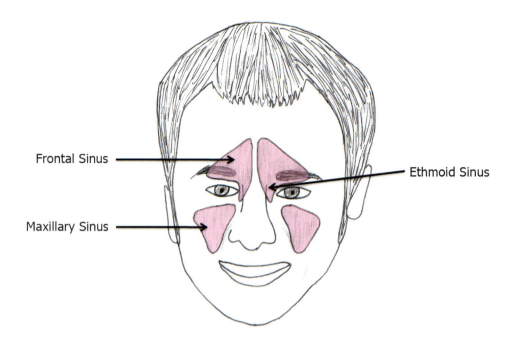

Maxillary Sinus — Largest paranasal sinus, located on both sides of the nose in the cheek area. Although they are rare tumors, maxillary sinus tumors account for the majority of all paranasal sinus tumors

- Signs and Symptoms
    - Tumor is generally silent until it extends beyond the sinus walls
    - Common symptoms include: nosebleeds, nasal obstructions, pain above or below the eyes, decreased sense of smell
- Most Common Histopathology
    - Squamous Cell Carcinoma
- Routes of Spread
    - Direct extension into the orbit (superior), oral cavity (inferior), nasal cavity (medial), and base of skull (posterior)
    - Lymph node drainage is rare in early stage carcinomas, but more extensive cancers commonly involve the jugulodigastric lymph node chain

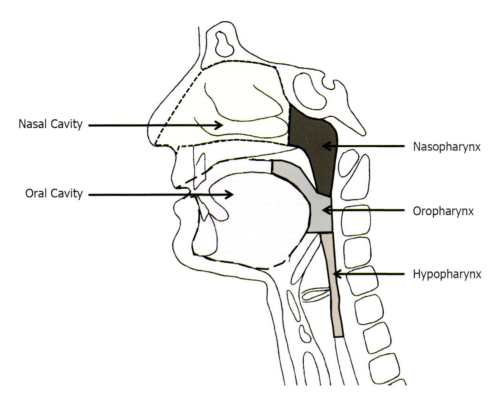

Oral Cavity – Consists of the lips (most common site of disease), floor of mouth, oral tongue, gingiva, hard palate, buccal mucosa, and retromolar trigone

- Signs and Symptoms
    - Chronic, non-healing ulcers, mouth pain, pre-malignant conditions (leukoplakia and erythroplasia)
- Most Common Histopathology
    - Squamous Cell Carcinoma
- Routes of Spread
    - Lip – Direct invasion
    - Floor of mouth/ Oral tongue – commonly present with submental and submandibular lymph node involvement

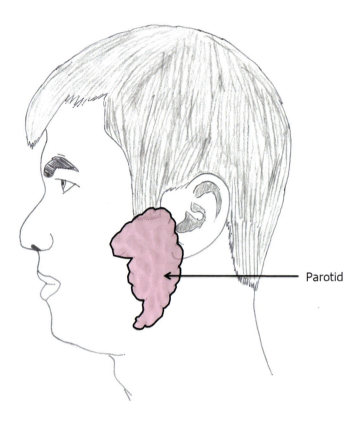

Parotid Gland – Largest of the salivary glands, it is L – shaped and located anterior and inferior to the ear. Most of the salivary tumors occur in the parotid. Parotid tumors can arise from metastatic skin cancer (more common than primary lesions)

- Signs and Symptoms
    - Mass or lump, pain, muscle weakness on one side of face
- Most Common Histopathology
    - Adenocarcinoma
- Routes of Spread
    - Most common spread is by local invasion (ipsilateral neck, lymph nodes, and perineural invasion)

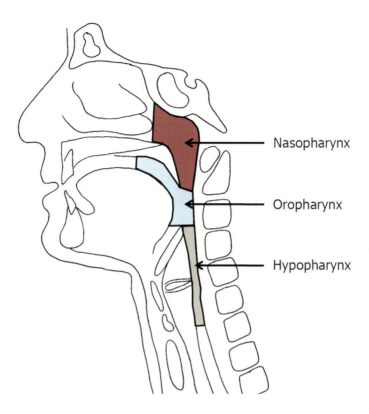

Nasopharynx – Located posterior to the soft palate with a rich lymphatic network.

- Signs and Symptoms

    o Mass or lump, hearing loss, ringing in the ear, feeling of fullness in the ear, nasal blockage, nosebleeds, headaches

- Most Common Histopathology

    o Squamous Cell Carcinoma

- Routes of Spread

    o Most commonly spreads to the lymphatics (80 – 90% of all tumors have cervical lymph node involvement)

- Treatment Options

    o Radiation therapy and chemotherapy are the most common treatments. New surgical techniques are developing to access nasopharyngeal tumors with less morbidity

Oropharynx – Includes the uvula, tonsillar fossae and pillars (most common site of disease), base of tongue, soft palate, and vallecula

- Signs and Symptoms
    - Painful swallowing, sore throat
- Most Common Histopathology
    - Squamous Cell Carcinoma
- Routes of Spread
    - Direct extension or lymphatic spread
        - Base of tongue – JD, submaxillary, and spinal accessory nodes
        - Tonsillar Fossae – JD and submaxillary nodes
        - Soft palate - JD, submaxillary, and spinal accessory nodes
        - Pharyngeal Wall – Retropharyngeal, pharyngeal, and JD nodes

Hypopharynx – Consists of the pyriform sinus (most common site of disease) and the posterior pharyngeal wall

- Signs and Symptoms
    - Dysphagia, painful neck nodes, mass or lump, ear pain
- Most Common Histopathology
    - Squamous Cell Carcinoma
- Routes of Spread
    - Hypopharynx has a rich lymphatic supply and tumors commonly have positive nodal spread to the jugulodigastric and midjugular nodes

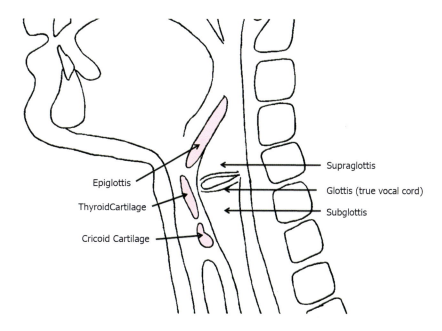

Larynx – The larynx extends from the tip of the epiglottis to the inferior border of the cricoid cartilage and is divided into three regions:

> Supraglottic – epiglottis, arytenoids, ventricle, false cord, and vestibule
>
> Glottic – true vocal cords
>
> Subglottic – Inferior to the true vocal cords (glottis)

- Signs and Symptoms
    - Hoarseness (most common in glottic tumors), sore throat, dysphagia
- Most Common Histopathology
    - Squamous Cell Carcinoma
- Routes of Spread
    - Supraglottic lesions present with nodal involvement in the JD and midjugular lymph nodes
    - Glottic lesions rarely spread due to lack of lymph nodes in the region. Prognosis of glottic cancers depends on the vocal cord fixation
    - Subglottic lesions spread to the peritracheal and cervical nodes
- Treatment Options
    - Early stage glottis lesions are cured with radiation therapy or surgery. Chemotherapy is not required unless the tumor is advanced

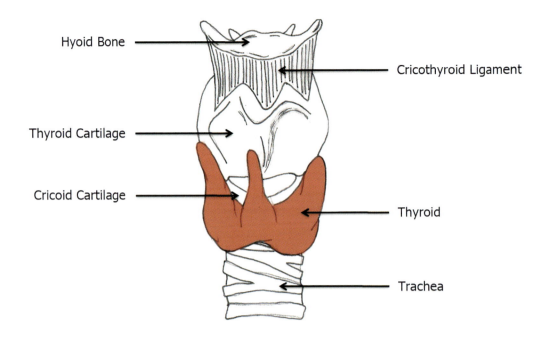

Thyroid – Aids the body in metabolism

Four types of thyroid neoplasms:

Papillary, follicular, medullary, and anaplastic

- Epidemiology and Etiology
    - Effects women more than men (All other head and neck cancers are more common in men)
- Signs and Symptoms
    - Rapid growth, pain or lump in neck
- Most Common Histopathology
    - Papillary tumors
- Routes of Spread
    - Papillary – Spread locally through the lymph nodes
    - Follicular – Blood born metastasis to liver, bone, and lung
- Treatment Options
    - Iodine-131, radioactive iodine (RAI) can be used after surgery to treat papillary or follicular thyroid cancers. Medullary tumors develop from C cells and do not take up RAI

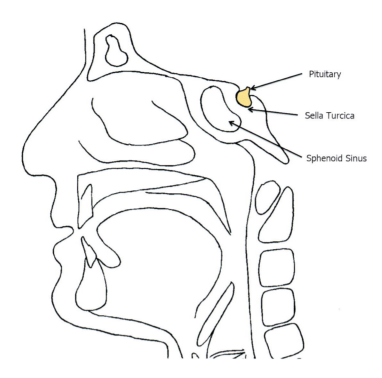

Pituitary –Regulates the activity of other glands in the body. Sits in the sella turcica, above the sphenoid sinus and inferior to the optic chiasm

- Epidemiology and Etiology

    o Multiple Endocrine Neoplasia, type 1 (MENS1) – hereditary condition that has a very high risk of developing tumors in the pituitary, parathyroid, and pancreas

- Signs and Symptoms

    o Endocrine problems, mass effects from the tumor (vision loss, headaches, intracranial pressure)

- Most Common Histopathology

    o Benign adenomas

- Routes of Spread

    o Histologically benign, does not spread through the lymphatics or blood. Can cause damage by local invasion and compression. Optic nerve compression can cause vision loss

- Treatment Options

    o Most pituitary tumors are benign. Observation, medications to control tumor growth, and surgery are the most common treatments. Radiation therapy may be used if medications fail to control tumor growth

Cancers in the Thorax

Organ	Tolerance Dose	End Point
Spinal Cord	4700 cGy	Necrosis
Esophagus	5500 cGy	Stricture/Perforation
Heart	4000 cGy	Pericarditis
Lung	1700 cGy	Pneumonitis
Brachial Plexus	5500 cGy	Nerve Damage

Thorax Radiation Side Effects

- Acute – Esophagitis, dermatitis, pneumonitis
- Chronic – Pneumonitis, fibrosis, esophageal stricture, pericarditis, heart problems

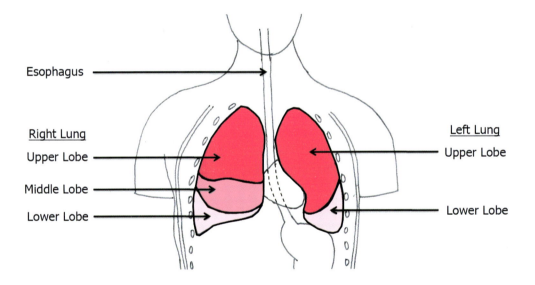

Lung – Respiratory organ

- Pleura – lining that surrounds the lungs
- Hilum – root of the lung at the right and left main stem bronchus
- Mediastinum – midline that separates the lungs. Composed of: heart, thymus, trachea, great vessels, esophagus, and lymph nodes

- Epidemiology and Etiology

    - Leading cause of cancer death in males and females
    - Common causes: Tobacco, asbestos, radon gas

- Signs and Symptoms
    - Most signs and symptoms do not appear until the cancer is in advanced stages
    - Cough that does not go away, chest pain, hoarseness, weight loss, loss of appetite, bloody sputum, shortness of breath, recurring chest infections, and a new onset of wheezing
- Most Common Histopathology
    - Two major types of lung cancer:
        - Small Cell – least common, but usually widespread by time of diagnosis
        - Non-small Cell - majority of lung cancers. 3 sub-types:
            Squamous cell
            Adenocarcinoma
            Large cell undifferentiated carcinoma
    - Mesotheliomas – rare, most common location is in the pleura of the lungs. Mesothelioma can also be found in the linings of other organs. Most common cause is asbestos exposure
    - Pancoast tumors (Superior sulcus tumor) - this tumor appears in the apex of the lung. The tumor can extend locally to involve the brachial plexus. Possible signs are: shoulder pain, muscle wasting, and rib destruction
        - Horner Syndrome – Nerve involvement from paravertebral tumor extension. Possible signs:
            Ptosis – drooping eyelids
            Meiosis – small pupils
            Anhydrosis – no sweat on affected side
- Treatment Options
    - Surgery, chemotherapy and radiation
        - Prophylactic Cranial Irradiation (PCI) – helps prevent brain metastasis for small cell carcinoma
        - HDR for endobronchial lesions and centrally located disease

Esophagus – muscular tube that carries food and liquid from the mouth to the stomach

- Epidemiology and Etiology

    o   More common in black men around 70 – 80 years old

    o   Common causes are tobacco and alcohol use, Barrett esophagus, and reflux disease

- Signs and Symptoms

    o   Weight loss, dysphagia, pain

    o   Signs of more advanced cancer: hoarseness, hiccups, pneumonia, high blood calcium levels

- Histopathology

    o   Adenocarcinoma – most commonly found in the lower part of the esophagus

    o   Squamous cell carcinoma – found anywhere in the esphagus

- Routes of Spread

    o   Tumor spread in the esophagus can skip sections of the esophagus causing "skip mets"

- Treatment Options

    o   Surgery, chemotherapy and radiation therapy. HDR can be used for accessible lesions

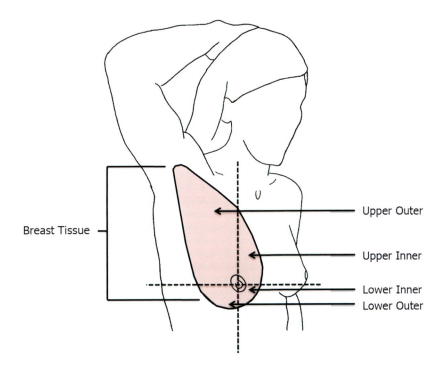

Breast – most common malignancy in women in the United States. The 2nd most common cancer death in women. Cancer is most often found in the upper-outer quadrant of the breast

Ductal carcinoma in situ is the most common type of non-invasive breast cancer. The stage is "0" because the cancer has not spread beyond the milk duct into the surrounding breast tissue

Lobular carcinoma in-situ originates in the lobules, the milk producing glands at the end of the milk ducts and is not considered a true cancer

- Epidemiology and Etiology
    - Personal or family history, $BRCA_1$ and $BRCA_2$ gene, history of atypical ductal hyperplasia, and nulliparity
- Signs and Symptoms
    - Lump or thickening of the breast found on self-exam or mammogram
    - Infammatory carcinoma – Breast appears erythematous, edematous, and indurated without palpable mass. Breast can be described as "peau d' orange" (French term meaning skin is dimpled in appearance)

- Most Common Histopathology

    - Infiltrating ductal carcinoma

- Routes of Spread

    - Axillary lymph nodes are most commonly involved, but lymph node spread depends on tumor location

    - The most common sites for metastatic spread are the bone, liver, lung, and brain

- Lymph Node assessment

    - Sentinel lymph node biopsy – uses dye or radioactive tracer to identify the first chain of lymph node drainage in the breast. If the node is positive to disease, a full axillary dissection can be done

    - Axillary lymph node dissection - total number of nodes involved correlate with prognosis and determine type of treatment

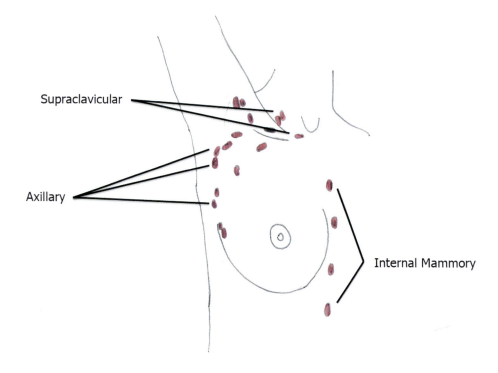

Abdominal Cancers

Pelvic and Whole Abdomen Radiation Side Effects

- Acute – Mucositis, erythema, diarrhea, nausea, vomiting, dysuria, proctitis, cystitis, and fatigue

- Chronic – Proctitis, enteritis, hemorrhagic cystitis, small bowel obstruction, vaginal adhesions, recto-vaginal fistula, and bowel perforation

Treatment Options

- Surgery, pre or post-operative radiation therapy, chemotherapy, brachytherapy

Routes of Spread

- Direct invasion, lymphatics, rarely blood

Mid-pelvic lesions

- Primary Nodes – Common iliac, internal iliac, external iliac

- Secondary Nodes – Periaortic

Low Lesions

- Primary Nodes – Inguinal

- Secondary Nodes – Internal iliac, external iliac, common iliac

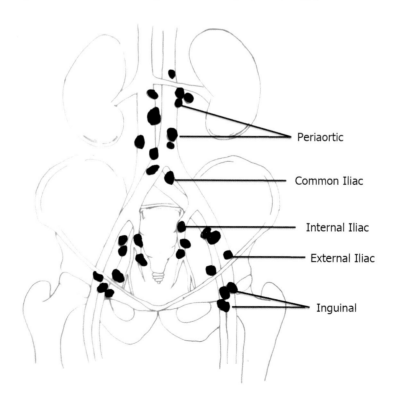

Organ	Tolerance Dose	Endpoint
Liver	3000 cGy	Liver Failure
Kidney	2300 cGy	Nephritis
Stomach	5500 cGy	Ulceration/Perforation
Spinal Cord	4700 cGy	Necrosis
Small Bowel	4500 cGy	Obstruction/Perforation
Large Bowel	5500 cGy	Obstruction/Perforation

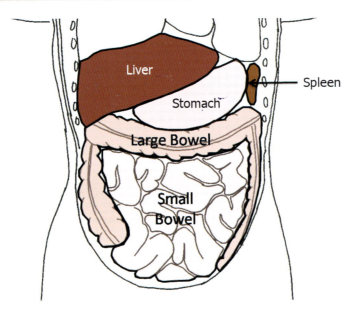

Pancreas —Endocrine and exocrine organ in the abdomen. Divided into 3 main sections: Head (where cancer most commonly develops), body, and tail. The pancreas is located inferior to the liver and posterior to the stomach

- Epidemiology and Etiology

    o Major risk factors include: smoking, chronic pancreatitis (inflammation of the pancreas associated with excessive alcohol intake or gallstones), diabetes mellitus, family history of pancreatic cancer

- Signs and Symptoms

    o Jaundice, pain

- Most Common Histopathology

    o Ductal adenocarcinoma

- Routes of Spread

    o Direct invasion, blood, lymphatics and peritoneal spread

Stomach - sac-like organ that holds food and begins the digestive process by secreting digestive gastric juices

- Signs and Symptoms
    - Weight loss, decreased appetite, abdominal pain, nausea, vomiting, heartburn like symptoms
- Most Common Histopathology
    - Adenocarcinoma
- Routes of Spread
    - Gastric cancers can spread by direct extension, and also through the rich lymphatic network

Pelvic Cancers

Organ	Tolerance Dose	End Point
Small Bowel	4500 cGy	Obstruction/Perforation
Large Bowel	5500 cGy	Obstruction/Perforation
Rectum	6000 cGy	Proctitis/Necrosis/Stenosis
Spinal Cord	4700 cGy	Necrosis
Kidney	2300 cGy	Nephritis
Liver	3000 cGy	Liver Failure
Femoral Head and Neck	5200 cGy	Necrosis
Bladder	6500 cGy	Contracture

Colorectal Cancer – Third most common cancer in men and women

- Epidemiology and Etiology
    - Family history, inflammatory bowel disease, polyps, diet low in fiber, high in fat
- Signs and Symptoms
    - Abdominal pain, melena (black, tarry stool), nausea, vomiting, change in bowel habits, tenesmus
- Most Common Histopathology
    - Adenocarcinoma
- Routes of Spread
    - Liver is the most common site for colorectal metastasis

- Treatment Options
    - Surgery, radiation therapy and chemotherapy
    - Surgical techniques
        - Anterior resection – remove colon, leave sphincter and rectum
        - Abdominoperineal resection (APR) – remove anus and part of rectum

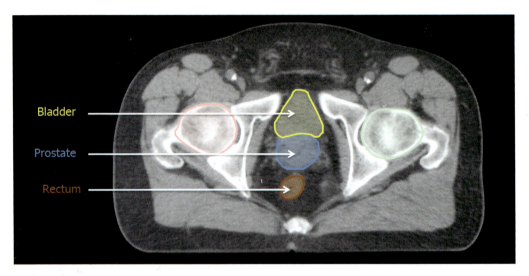

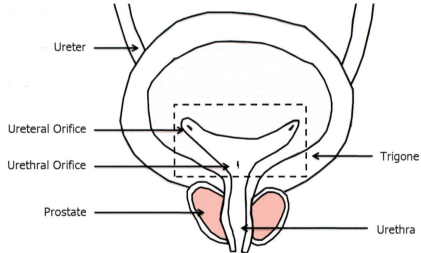

Bladder – The trigone of the bladder is the most common site for bladder cancers. The trigone is the area of the bladder formed by two ureters posteriolaterally and the urethral orifice anteriorly

- Epidemiology and Etiology
    - Smoking, chronic bladder irritations (indwelling catheters)

- Signs and Symptoms
    - Early stage cancers may or may not have symptoms
    - Hematuria, hesitancy, dysuria
- Most Common Histopathology
    - Urothelial (transitional cell)
- Treatment Options
    - Surgery, chemotherapy and radiation therapy

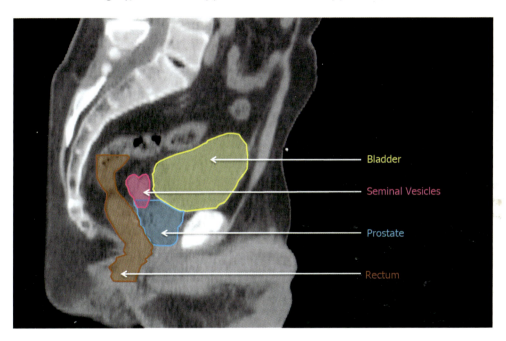

Prostate – Located inferior to the bladder and anterior to the rectum in males. Prostate cancer usually originates in the periphery of the gland. (Benign Prostatic Hypertrophy (BPH) begins centrally, around the urethra) There are normally multiple foci of the tumor

- Epidemiology and Etiology
    - Most common cancer in males (excluding skin cancer)
    - 2nd leading cause of cancer death in males
    - Associated with high fat intake and high testosterone levels
- <u>Signs and Symptoms</u>
    - Early stage cancers may not have symptoms

- o Symptoms include: blood in urine, impotence, nocturia, hesitancy, firm nodule on rectal exam, elevated PSA (prostate specific antigen), pain in pelvis, spine, hips, or ribs

- Most Common Histopathology
  - o Adenocarcinoma

- Routes of Spread
  - o <u>Bone</u> is the most common metastatic site for prostate cancer

- Grading
  - o Gleason score is used to grade prostate carcinomas. Multiple biopsies are taken from the prostate and they are graded from 1 to 5 (5 being the worst prognosis). The two worst grades are added and together make up the Gleason score (Gleason sum)

- Diagnostic Studies
  - o Biopsy is used to rule out BPH
  - o PSA is a protein released by normal and malignant prostate tissue. PSA is a tumor marker and is used to predict prognosis before treatment and is also used to follow up after treatment
  - o An elevation in PSA may indicate tumor recurrence

Testicular – external male organs responsible for producing sperm and testosterone. The testicles form near the 2nd lumbar vertebrae and later descend into the scrotal sac. There are two main types of testicular cancers, seminomas and non-seminomas. Seminomas are less common and are slow growing. Non-seminomas are more common and grow quickly. Both types originate in the germ cells

- Epidemiology and Etiology
  - o Most common cancer in men between the ages 20 and 34
  - o Accounts for 1% of cancer in males and is one of the most curable

- Signs and Symptoms
  - o Usually presents as a painless swelling in the scrotum (testicular mass)
  - o Later stage cancers can present with back pain and abdominal swelling

- Most Common Histopathology
  - o Germ Cell

- Routes of Spread
    - Pure seminomas have a tendency to remain localized or only involve lymphatics
    - Non-seminomas more frequently spread by blood
- Treatment Options
    - The most common treatment for seminoma and non-seminoma is surgery to remove the testicle. Non-seminoma may require chemotherapy. Seminomas may be treated with chemotherapy and/or radiation therapy. Seminomas are very radiosensitive. Daily radiation dose and total prescribed dose are generally lower than standard fractionation

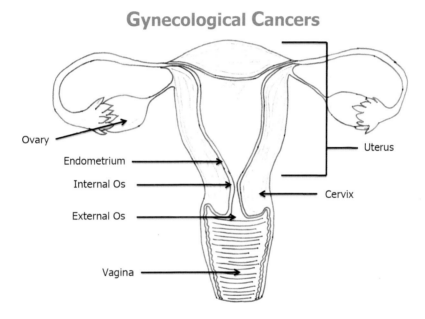

Cervix – Lower 1/3 of the uterus

- Epidemiology and Etiology
    - Human Papilloma Virus (HPV) is the most common risk factor
    - Early age intercourse, large number of pregnancies
    - 35 – 55 years old
    - Carcinoma in-situ is four times more common than invasive carcinoma
    - The pap smear has helped to lower death rates significantly
- Signs and Symptoms
    - Increased menstrual bleeding, foul smelling discharge, bleeding following intercourse, pain, and urinary and rectal symptoms in late stages

- Most Common Histopathology
    - Squamous Cell Carcinoma
- Routes of Spread
    - Direct extension and lymphatics
    - Barrel lesions – Barrel lesions are bulky tumors of the endocervix that are over 4 cm in diameter. They have a worse prognosis, even when localized due to the large tumor mass

Endometrium

There are three layers of the uterus

Endometrium – Inner mucus membrane layer

Myometrium – Smooth muscle layer

Perimetrium – Outer serous coat

- Epidemiology and Etiology
    - Endometrial cancer is the <u>most common</u> invasive GYN cancer
    - Obesity, nulliparity, infertility, hypertension, early menarchy, and late menopause
- Signs and Symptoms
    - Unusual spotting, bleeding, or discharge, pelvic pain or mass
- Most Common Histopathology
    - Squamous Cell Carcinoma
- Diagnostic Studies
    - Dilation and Curettage (D&C) is the most definitive method of diagnosis

Ovarian – almond shaped bodies attached to both sides of the uterus. Their function is to produce an egg (ova) and two hormones (estrogen and progesterone). The ovaries are attached to the uterus by the utero-ovarian ligament

- Epidemiology and Etiology
    - Most common cause of GYN cancer death (rarely found in early stages)
    - Common causes: Nulliparity, infertility, family history, estrogen and hormone replacement therapy

- Signs and Symptoms
    - Back pain (most common), fatigue, bloating, constipation, abdominal pain, and urinary frequency
    - Later symptoms include: swelling of the abdomen, cramping, pressure, vaginal bleeding, and back pain
- Most Common Histopathology
    - Epithelial
- Treatment Options
    - Surgery and chemotherapy are the most common treatment for ovarian cancer. Radiation therapy is rarely used due to potential spread in the lining of the abdomen (peritoneum), and the inability to effectively treat the entire abdomen to an adequate dose

Vagina and Vulva

Vagina – musculomembranous tube that forms a passageway from the vulva to the uterus

Vulva – female external genitalia

- Epidemiology and Etiology
    - Very rare cancers, associated with smoking and HPV
- Signs and Symptoms
    - Vagina – Bleeding, discharge, mass, pain during intercourse, painful urination
    - Vulva – Red, white, or pink bumps, itching, bleeding, discharge
- Most Common Histopathology
    - Squamous Cell Carcinoma

Cancer of the Lymphatic System

Lymphoma – There are two types of malignant lymphomas: Hodgkin and Non-Hodgkin (NHL). These two lymphomas are distinguished by microscopic inspection

Chemotherapy and Radiation Side Effects

- Chemotherapy – hair loss, mouth sores, suppressed immune system, bruising, bleeding, and fatigue. Long term side effects – sterility

- Radiation therapy
    - Early – hair loss, sore throat, skin erythema, dysphagia
    - Late – pneumonitis, hypothyroidism, herpes zoster, Lhermittes sign
- Epidemiology and Etiology
    - Hodgkin – Occurs in two age groups (bimodal), 15-40 years old and over 55. Overall survival rate is around 90% due to advanced treatment techniques
    - Non-Hodgkin (NHL) – Survival rates for NHL vary based on location, stage, and subtype of the disease. NHL is more common in the 40 to 70 year old range.
- Signs and Symptoms
    - Painless swelling of nodes, fever, drenching night sweats, weight loss (10% body weight in 6 months), fatigue, coughing or breathing problems (from mediastinal node involvement)
- Most Common Histopathology
    - Hodgkin – the diagnostic cell is the Reed-Sternberg cell. This cell contains two nuclei with prominent nucleoli. Pathological type determines prognosis
    - Non-Hodgkin – two main types of lymphocytes that develop in to lymphomas:
        - B-type lymphocytes (B cells) – most common
        - T-lymphocytes (T cells)
- Staging
    - Ann Arbor staging is the most common staging system for lymphomas
- Treatment Options
    - The most common treatments are combinations of chemotherapy and radiation therapy. Lymphomas are very chemosensitive and radiosensitive
    - Bone marrow transplants may be used for patients when other treatment options are not successful

Cancers of the Central Nervous System

Radiation Side Effects – Radiation necrosis (occurs months to years after radiation from the irradiation of normal cells), fatigue, headache, edema, hair loss, and changes in brain function (usually with large areas of radiation)

Organ	Tolerance Dose	End Point
Brain (limited)	6000 cGy	Necrosis/Infarction
Brain (whole)	4500 cGy	Necrosis/Infarction
Brain Stem	5000 cGy	Necrosis/Infarction
Optic Nerve	5000 cGy	Blindness
Retina	4500 cGy	Blindness
Ear	3000 cGy/5500 cGy	Acute/Chronic Serous Otitis
Spinal Cord	4700 cGy	Necrosis

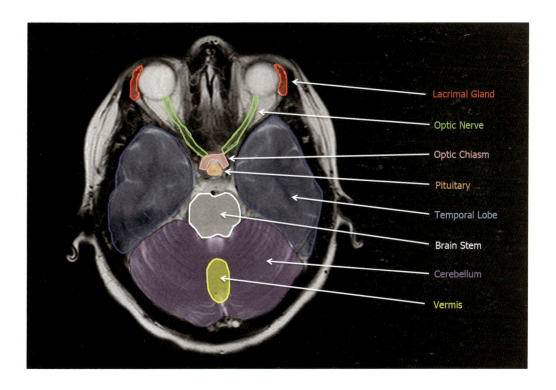

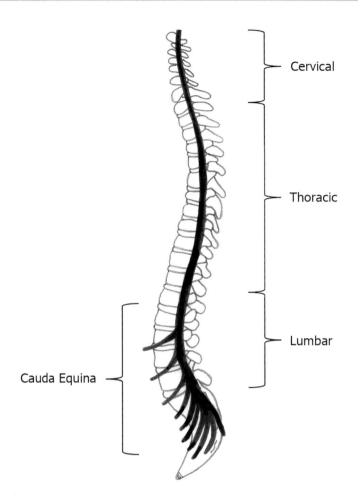

Spinal Cord – The spinal cord starts in the brain (medulla) and ends at approximately L1-L2 in adults. The spinal cord does not extend the entire length of the spinal column. A nerve bundle called the cauda equina starts at approximately at L1 and ends at the coccyx

- Epidemiology and Etiology

    o Most spinal cord tumors originate outside the dura mater (extra dural) and are metastatic. Intra dural spine tumors are primary spinal tumors and are rare

- Signs and Symptoms

    o Pain and weakness are the most common symptoms. Other symptoms include sensory changes and sphincter dysfunction

- Treatment Options

    o A spinal cord compression constitutes an emergency. Radiation therapy may be initiated immediately to reduce the possibility of further damage. The dose for an emergency treatment is generally a higher daily dose for the first 2 or 3 treatments

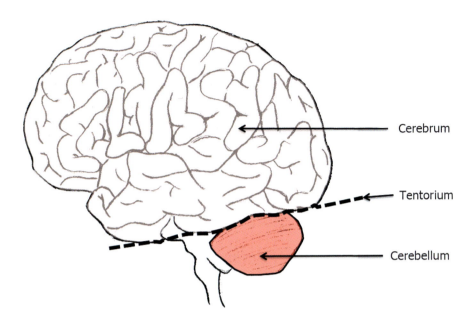

Brain – the tentorium cerebelli is an extension of the dura mater and divides the cerebrum and cerebellum. Adult brain tumors are more common above the tentorium, and children's brain tumors are more common below the tentorium

Primary Brain Tumors – the most common primary brain tumors are gliomas which include the two most common types of tumor, astrocytoma and glioblastoma multiforme. The grade of the tumor is the most important predictor for survival. High grade tumors are more aggressive and are associated with lower survival rates

- Astrocytoma – the most common type of brain tumor in children, originates in the brainstem, cerebellum, white matter of the cerebrum, or spinal cord

- Glioblastoma Multiforme (GBM) – most common type of brain tumor in adults, originates in the glial cells in the cerebrum. This is a high grade tumor with a poor prognosis

- Brainstem Glioma – originates in the medulla, pons, or midbrain. Difficult to biopsy due to bad location. Overall bad prognosis

- Schwannoma – originates in the Schwann cells which surround the cranial nerves and other nerves responsible for hearing and balance. Usually benign

- Ependymoma – originates in the ependymal cells which line the ventricles. May block the exit of cerebrospinal fluid causing the ventricles to enlarge (hydrocephalus). Does not spread or infiltrate normal brain tissue. Sometimes curable by surgery. Average age is 21 years old

- Medulloblastoma – second most common type of brain tumor in children. Originates in the fourth cerebral ventricle and the cerebellum, and often invades the meninges. (the cerebellum controls coordination)

- Oligodendroglioma – originates in the brain cells called oligodendrocytes. These are benign, slow growing tumors and usually occur in the frontal lobe. In most cases, the entire tumor cannot be removed with surgery and radiation therapy is used for residual disease

Secondary (metastatic) Brain Tumors – these tumors are more common than primary brain tumors. In adults, the most common type of cancers that spread to the brain are: lung, breast, melanomas, and cancers of the gastrointestinal tract

- Signs and Symptoms
    - Symptoms are often caused from increased pressure in the skull such as: headache, nausea, vomiting, and blurred vision
    - Tumor location correlates with presenting symptoms (e.g. a tumor in the cerebellum can affect coordination)
- Routes of Spread
    - Primary tumors of the CNS rarely spread outside the central nervous system. They can spread by local invasion and cerebrospinal fluid seeding
- Treatment Options
    - Surgery, Radiation Therapy and Chemotherapy
    - There is a blood brain barrier between the brain and the vascular system of the CNS, chemotherapeutic drugs are sometimes blocked from passing this blood brain barrier. Radiation can be used to control disease in the brain
    - Corticosteroids such as decadron are used to reduce cerebral edema

Solid Tumors of Childhood

Wilms tumor – Nephroblastoma

- Epidemiology and Etiology
    - The most common renal tumor in children, usually occurs between the ages of 2 and 5 years old
- Signs and Symptoms
    - Asymptomatic flank or abdominal mass, pain, hematuria, and increased blood pressure
- Most Common Histopathology
    - Favorable histology

- Routes of Spread
  - Lung is the most common site of metastasis
- Treatment Options
  - Surgery and chemotherapy are the most common treatments. Radiation therapy is used for unfavorable histology and advanced stages

Rhabdomyosarcoma – most common soft tissue sarcoma under the age of 15. Can arise anywhere in the body, is locally invasive, and disseminates early

- Routes of Spread
  - Relapse is dictated by the routes of spread via blood and lymphatics. Relapse is usually local, but distant sites of metastasis include: lung, CNS, lymph nodes, liver, bone marrow, and soft tissue

Leukemia

Cancer of the blood forming cells. Leukemia starts in the bone marrow but usually spreads quickly through the blood. Over time, leukemia spreads to lymph nodes, spleen, liver, the covering of the brain and spinal cord, spinal fluid, and other organs

There are four major types of leukemia which are grouped by the type of cell affected and the rate of cell growth:

- Acute Lymphocytic Leukemia (ALL) – cancer is formed in the bone marrow cells that form lymphocytes (lymphoblasts (immature cells)). This leukemia progresses rapidly without treatment
- Acute Myelogenous Leukemia (AML) – cancer is formed in the bone marrow cells that form red blood cells, some white blood cells, and platelets (myeoblasts (immature cells)). This leukemia progresses rapidly without treatment
- Chronic Lymphocytic Leukemia (CLL) – cancer is formed in the lymphocytes. These non-functioning cells replace normal cells in the bone marrow and lymph nodes, weakening the patients' immune response. These cells crowd out normal red blood cells, white blood cells, and platelets. Some patients have slight symptoms that do not require treatment for long periods of time
- Chronic Myelogenous Leukemia (CML) – cancer is formed in the myelocytes. This disease can progress slowly over years without symptoms or treatment. Eventually the abnormal cells cause symptoms due to the lack of normal red blood cells, white blood cells, and platelets

Acute leukemias usually show more dramatic remission and survival benefits than chronic leukemias. Chronic leukemias are generally less fatal and have a more prolonged course without therapy

- Epidemiology and Etiology
    - Leukemia can occur at any age, but it is more common in people over 60 years old
    - The most common types of leukemia in adults are: AML and CLL
    - Leukemia is the most common cancer in children and adolescents and the most common type of leukemia in children is ALL
- Signs and Symptoms
    - Fatigue, lack of appetite, paleness of skin (due to anemia), infection, fever that does not improve, bleeding, bruising, bone pain, swelling of abdomen, and swollen lymph nodes
- Diagnostic Tests
    - Bone marrow aspiration and biopsy, lumbar puncture (spinal tap)
- Treatment Options
    - The most effective form of treatment is chemotherapy, but a blood stem cell transplant can also be performed
    - Biological therapy can also be used (growth factors, interleukins, monoclonal antibodies)

Sarcomas

There are two types of sarcomas: Soft tissue sarcoma, and bone sarcoma. Sarcomas commonly metastasize to lung, lymphatics are rarely involved

Soft Tissue Sarcoma –develop from connective tissue: muscle, tendon, fat, fibrous, and synovial tissues. Very rare tumors (less than 1% of all cancers) Most often found in muscle groups and is usually confined to the muscle compartments. Can spread up to 10 centimeters longitudinally in the muscle compartment

- Most common sites
    - Adults – extremities (most commonly the thigh because of increased muscle mass)
    - Children – trunk (retroperitoneum, mediastinum, chest wall, abdomen, breast), head, or neck

- Most Common Histopathology (subtypes)
    - Liposarcomas (fat)
    - Leiomyosarcomas (smooth muscle)
    - Rhabdomyosarcomas (striated muscle)
    - Malignant fibrous histiocytomas (mixed fiberblasts and other cells)
- Grading
    - Histological grade is the most important prognostic factor
- Treatment Options
    - Surgery, Chemotherapy and Radiation Therapy

Bone Tumors

- <u>Primary</u> - Not as common as metastatic lesions. Spreads through the bloodstream. The most common metastatic site is the lungs
    - Osteosarcoma – most common bone tumor in children and adolescents. More likely to occur in males and forms in the arms, legs, and pelvis. This tumor is radioresistant
    - Ewing Sarcoma – second most common bone tumor in children. Most often found in the diaphysis of long bones in the lower body. More responsive to radiation than osteosarcoma
    - Chondrosarcoma – composed of cartilaginous elements. Second most common primary bone tumor and can occur at any age (most commonly over 20 years old.) The most common site of disease is in the pelvis
    - Multiple Myeloma – non-osseous bone tumor. Osteolytic (dark holes) on x-ray because bone is eaten away. Multiple myeloma develops in the plasma cells of bone marrow. Incidence increases with age. Symptoms are bone pain, bleeding, infections, and renal failure
- <u>Metastatic</u> – most common bone tumors. Occur most frequently in the spine and pelvis

Skin Cancer

Skin cancer is the most common type of cancer (>50%), and commonly presents in the head and neck area. There are two major divisions of skin cancer: Non-melanoma and melanoma

<u>Non-melanoma</u> – Includes all skin cancers except malignant melanomas. There are 2 main types of non-melanoma skin cancers:

- Basal Cell Carcinoma (BCCA) – the tumors arise from the deepest layer of the dermis called the basal layer and make up a majority of all skin cancers. These cancers normally spread by direct invasion, lymphatic spread is rare. BCCA is most commonly found in the head and neck area above a line drawn from the corner of the mouth to the ear lobe

- Squamous Cell Carcinoma (SCCA) – develops in the more superficial layers of the epidermis and commonly appears on sun exposed areas. These tumors are more aggressive than BCCA, and can invade surrounding tissue and spread to the lymphatics

- Signs and Symptoms
    - New growth, enlarged spot or lump, and a sore that does not heal

- Treatment Options
    - Moh's surgery – successive biopsies are performed and examined under a microscope until margins are clear. Surgery offers a rapid cure without the side effects of radiation
    - Radiation therapy provides a high cure rate and preserves function with good cosmesis
    - Topical chemotherapy

Melanoma – originates from the melanocytes. Melanomas are less common than BCCA and SCCA, but far more aggressive. Melanomas start superficial but spread deep, and can be spread by lymphatics and blood. The most common site for metastasis is the lungs. Prognosis is determined by the depth of invasion using Breslow or Clark staging

Less Common Skin Cancers

- Kaposi Sarcoma – tumors below the skin surface that appear as raised, red, purple, or brown blotches. Common in HIV patients as well as Jewish and Mediterranean men

- Mycosis Fungoides – type of Non-Hodgkin Lymphoma and is the most common form of cutaneous T cell lymphoma. Affects the skin but may progress internally over time
    - Treatment Options
        - Surgery, Chemotherapy and Radiation Therapy

Benign Skin Lesions

- Keloid– benign, raised overgrowths of scar tissue that occur at the site of skin injury. Keloids must first be removed by surgery and then treated with radiation (electrons or superficial) soon after surgery to prevent the regrowth of scar tissue

Cancers of the Eyes

Benign Ocular Diseases

- Pterygium – fibrovascular proliferation of the conjunctiva. This is the most common benign ocular condition which radiation is beneficial. Pterygium is removed first by surgery and followed up with post operative radiation using a Strontium-90 or Yttrium-90 beta-emitting applicator to reduce recurrence rates

- Graves Ophthalmology – In some patients with hyperthyroidism, exopthalmos (anterior bulging of the eye) can occur. The primary tissues involved are the extraocular muscles. Radiation can be used when there is an optic nerve compression, but steroids are the first line of treatment

Malignant Eye Tumors

Retinoblastomas – most common intraocular malignancy of childhood. This tumor originates from the photoreceptor cells. Some retinoblastomas are inherited (gene mutation). Inherited retinoblastomas usually occur at a younger age

- Signs and Symptoms
    - Leukocoria (white pulpillary reflex), strabismus (squint), and mass in fundus

- Routes of Spread
    - Direct extension, lymphatics and bloodstream

- Treatment Options
    - Unilateral disease – enucleation
    - Bilateral disease - enucleation for eye with advanced disease, radiation therapy for the other eye
    - Chemotherapy for advanced disease

Radiation Protection and Quality Assurance

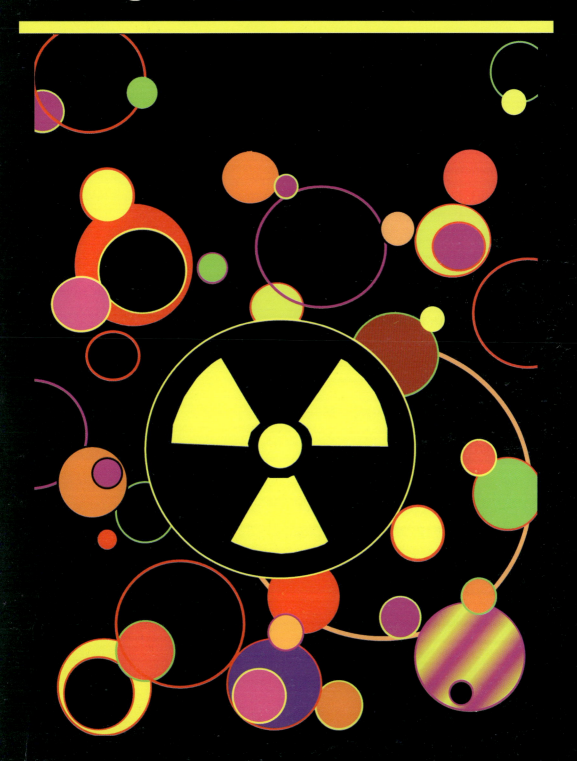

Radiation Physics and Biology

Sources of Radiation

- Natural background radiation
    - Cosmic Rays
    - Terrestrial radiation
    - Internal

Radioactive Isotopes (Brachytherapy)

Isotope	Half Life	Clinical Use	Radiation Type
Iodine- 125	59.4 days	LDR prostate	Permanent Implant
Palladium- 103	17 days	LDR prostate	Permanent Implant
Cesium- 137	30 years	LDR GYN	Temporary Implant
Iridium- 192	73.8 days	HDR prostate, breast, lung, GYN	Temporary Implant
Strontium- 90	28.8 days	Pterygium	Temporary Contact
Iodine- 131	8 days	Thyroid treatment	Ingested

Clinical Radiation Generators

- Kilovoltage Units
    - Superficial (≈50-150 KV)
    - Orthovoltage (≈150-500 KV)
- Megavoltage Units
    - Linear Accelerator (photons and electrons)
    - Cyclotron (Particle Therapy)
    - Cobalt-60 (Gamma rays)

Types of Radiation

Alpha Particles (α)

- Helium nucleus (2 protons and 2 neutrons)
- Emitted from an unstable nucleus
- Travels short distances
- Produces intense ionizations- High Linear Energy Transfer (LET)
- Extremely hazardous if ingested or inhaled

Beta Particles (β)

- Electrons emitted by the nucleus
- Shielded with low Z materials
- More penetrating than alpha

    B- Decay (Negatron)

    - Unstable nucleus with high neutron to proton ratio
    - Neutron converted to a proton, electron, and an antineutrino
        - Antineutrino – Small particle (no mass, no charge)

    B+ Decay (Positron)

    - Unstable nucleus with high proton to neutron ratio
    - Proton converted to neutron, positron, and neutrino
        - Neutrino – Small particle (no mass, no charge)
        - Positron – Combines with electron and annihilates (Unstable)

    X-ray and Gamma Ray (γ) (Photons)

Electromagnetic Radiation

- Frequency- Number of waves that pass a given point in a specified unit of time. The unit is Hertz (cycles/second)
- Wavelength- Distance between peaks of the wave, measured in meters
- Energy (E)=hv
    - v= frequency
    - h= Plank's Constant (6.62×10^{-34})
- Shorter Wavelength= greater energy and penetrating power
- Photons have no mass, no charge, and low LET

    Gamma Rays – emitted from the nucleus

    X-Rays – emitted from outside the nucleus

X-ray Beam Quality

The penetrating ability of the beam

- Half Value Layer (HVL) is the thickness of a given material that reduces the intensity of the radiation beam by one half

- X-ray beam **quality** increases (scatter radiation is reduced) with half value layer thickness (beam hardening)

- Attenuation equation = $I_x = I_o e^{-\mu x}$

    - I_o = incident beam intensity
    - I_x = exiting beam intensity
    - e = constant (2.718...)
    - µ = linear attenuation coefficient
        - function of absorber material and beam energy
        - decreases with increasing energy
    - x = absorber thickness

- The attenuation equation is used to calculate beam intensities for various absorber thicknesses

- If an incident energy of 1 and a transmitted energy of 0.5 (50%) is substituted into the attenuation equation, the HVL (x) multiplied by the linear attenuation coefficient must equal 0.693 because 0.693 is the exponent value that gives a final value of 0.5, or half the remaining intensity

$$I = I_o e^{-\mu x}$$

$$0.5 = 1.0 e^{-\mu x}$$

- The HVL is inversely proportional to the attenuation coefficient

$$HVL = \frac{0.693}{\mu}$$

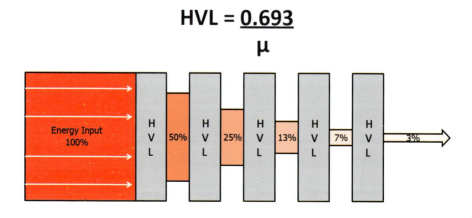

Monochromatic vs. Polychromatic Radiation

Monochromatic

- All photons in the radiation beam have the same energy

Polychromatic

- Photons in beam have varying energies
- An absorber removes lower energy X-rays
- Attenuation of polychromatic radiation results in:
    - Change in beam quantity (fewer photons)
    - Change in beam quality (lower energy photons are removed from the beam- beam hardening)
- Higher energy (hard) beams have:
    - Higher Half Value Layer
    - Higher penetrating power
- Lower energy (soft) beams have:
    - Lower Half Value Layer
    - Less penetrating power
    - Higher skin dose

Photon Interactions with Matter

Photoelectric Effect

- Transfer of total energy of a photon to an inner electron of an atom
- Photon interacts with an inner shell (K or L) and ejects an electron from the atom (ionization). The photon disappears
- An electron from an outer shell fills the vacancy and gives off characteristic radiation
- The photoelectric effect is more common with low energy photons and high atomic number (Z) materials, such as bone. The probability is proportional to Z^3 and inversely proportional to the energy ($1/energy^3$). As energy increases, the probability of this interaction decreases

Compton Scatter

- Photons interact with an outer shell (loosely bound) electron, the atom absorbs all the photon energy and the electron is ejected from the outer shell
- Compton scatter is the dominant interaction in soft tissue with photons in diagnostic and therapeutic energy ranges
- Most common interaction with the energies used in radiation therapy

Pair Production

- High energy photon interacts with the nucleus
- Incoming photon must have an energy of at least 1.02 MeV (threshold)
- Photon energy creates mass of negative and positive (positron) electrons, photon disappears
- When the positron stops, it undergoes annihilation and creates two .51 MeV photons traveling in opposite directions

Electron Interactions with Matter

Bremsstrahlung Radiation

- "Braking Radiation"
- Interaction of a charged particle (electron) with the nucleus of an atom
- The particle loses speed and changes direction
- The kinetic energy lost by the particle is emitted as bremsstrahlung radiation

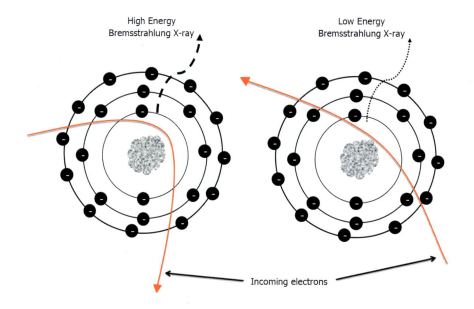

Characteristic Radiation

- Photon interacts with inner shell electron, ejecting it from the atom (ionization)

- An electron from an outer shell jumps to fill the vacancy and yields characteristic radiation equal to the element's electron binding energy

- The energy given off identifies the element. The radiation given off is *characteristic* of that element

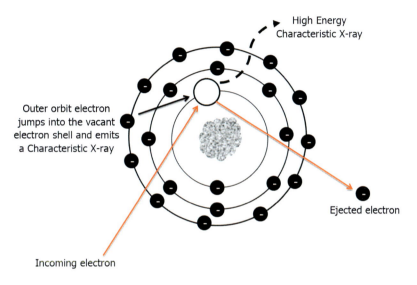

Radiation Energy Transfer

- Linear Energy Transfer (LET) - Rate that energy is deposited as it travels through matter

- Low LET – x and gamma rays, secondary electrons: small particles travel great distance

- High LET – protons, alpha particles: bulky particles travel small distance

    o Cell survival curve - shoulder region decreased or absent

    o Steeper curve

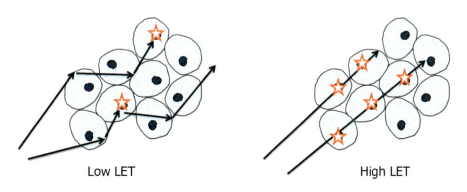

Radiation Interactions

- Direct Ionizations are more prominent with charged particles such as protons and electrons
    - Particles interact with the nucleus of an atom causing damage to the DNA of the cell. The DNA is the "target" for the radiation and a direct hit will kill the cell
- Indirect Ionizations are usually caused by x-rays, gamma rays, and neutrons
- These cause secondary effects within the cells
    - Radiolysis- splitting of a water molecule to form ions
    - Ions can recombine to form water and cause no damage or they can form damaging ions such as hydrogen peroxide which interact with the cellular components

Biological Effects of Radiation

- Low dose rates are less efficient in producing damage than high dose rates
- An organ's response to radiation is a function of:
    - Dose (rate and number of fractions)
    - Volume irradiated
    - Time of observation after irradiation
    - The most sensitive cell in the organ

General Side Effects of Radiation

- Early (Acute) Effects- observable within a period of hours to weeks
    - Nausea
    - Hair Loss (epilation) 1000 cGy temporary hair loss, 4000 – 4500 cGy permanent hair loss
    - Fatigue
    - Low Blood count due to bone marrow exposure and lymphocyte damage
        - Lymphocytes are extremely sensitive to radiation
    - Skin erythema begins at doses of 300 cGy-1000 cGy (standard fractionation) and progresses to dry desquamation and to moist desquamation

- Gonadal Dysfunction- 300 cGy temporary sterility, 1500 – 2000 cGy permanent sterility
- Chromosomal aberrations

- Late (Chronic) Effects- observable within a period of months to years
  - Scarring-radiation causes increased connective tissue, fibrosis, and scarring
  - Genetic Effects- Exposure of reproductive organs increases the risk of abnormal mutations and genetic changes
  - Carcinogenicity- Radiation can cause cancer
  - Leukemia-20 year risk post-radiation, peak incidence is 5-7 years
  - Other malignancies- Solid tumors
    - Thyroid, bone, lung, and breast cancers
  - General life span shortening
  - Genetic damage
  - Cataract Formation- latent period of 15 years

Effects of Whole Body Radiation Exposure

Radiation Syndromes

- Hematopoietic Syndrome
  - Dose- 200 – 1000 cGy (whole body) *2-10 Gy*
  - Mean Survival- 10 – 60 days
  - Symptoms – Nausea, vomiting, diarrhea, anemia, leukopenia, hemorrhage, fever, infection, and dehydration
  - Cause of death – Infection and dehydration

- Gastrointestinal Syndrome
  - Dose- 1000 – 5000 cGy (whole body) *10-50 Gy*
  - Mean Survival - 4-10 days
  - Symptoms – Same as hematopoietic plus electrolyte imbalance, lethargy, fatigue, and shock
  - Cause of death- Severe damage to the lining of the intestines

- Central Nervous System Syndrome

    - Dose – 2000 – 5000 cGy (whole body)
    - Mean Survival – 0 -3 days
    - Symptoms – Same as gastrointestinal plus ataxia, edema, vasculitis, and meningitis
    - Cause of death – Edema of the brain

General Effects of Whole Body Radiation

- Hematologic Depression- 25 cGy
- Death- Lethal Dose (LD) 50/30: Fifty percent of the population will die within 30 days with whole body doses of approximately 450 cGy

Radiation Protection

The goal of radiation protection is to prevent the occurrence of serious radiation induced complications and limit stochastic effects to a reasonable level

- Stochastic Effects – the probability of an effect rather than the severity of an effect. Stochastic effects are functions of radiation dose without thresholds (cancer and genetic effects)
- Non Stochastic (deterministic) effects – the severity of the effect varies with the radiation dose. Non stochastic effects have threshold doses (cataract formation and erythema)

Standards/ Recommendations/ Regulations from the NRC and NCRP

- NCRP – The National Council on Radiation Protection and Measurements is a group of technical experts who make recommendations on radiation protection and units. The NCRP are not a law making government agency, but their recommendations are usually adopted as law
- NRC – The Nuclear Regulatory Commission determines what will be law for many radiation concerns, not just radiation protection. These laws are listed in the Code of Federal Regulations (CFR) and are usually based on NCRP recommendations. States may be NRC regulated or Agreement States. Agreement States make their own regulations, but they must be as stringent as the NCR laws

The following recommendations exclude any exposure from personal medical procedures

NCRP #116 – 1993

Occupational Dose Limits:

Whole Body (stochastic)	50 mSv/year (5 rem/year)
Cumulative Effective Dose Limit	10 mSv X age (1 rem X age)
Lens of Eye (deterministic)	150 mSv/year (15 rem/year)
Skin, Hands, and Feet (deterministic)	500 mSv/year (50 rem/year)

Public Dose Limits (stochastic):

| Public Dose Limit | 1 mSv/year (.1 rem/year) |
| Embryo-Fetus (after declaration) | .5 mSv/month (.05 rem/month) |

Code of Federal Regulations (CFR) – NRC Regulations

CFR 10, parts 20 and 35

Occupational Dose Limits:

Total Effective Dose Equivalent (Deep and organ dose)	5 rem/year
Eye Dose Equivalent	15 rem/year
Shallow Dose Equivalent (Skin or extremity)	50 rem/year

Public Dose Limits

General Public	.1 rem/year
Minors	10% of dose to adult workers
Embryo-Fetus (after declaration)	.5 rem/pregnancy

Records of Accumulated Dose

- State and federal regulations require monitoring of anyone who may receive 10% of the Maximum Permissible Dose (MPD)

- When occupationally exposed workers change employment, exposure records should be transferred to the new employer

- Institutions must keep exposure records indefinitely

Monitoring for Radiation Protection

- Employees in the field of radiation must be monitored for accumulated absorbed dose during their time of employment (personnel monitors). Monitors are also used to survey a room for a radioactive substance and to verify radiation treatment standards (area monitors)

Monitoring Device	Description/Uses
TLD Badges	Thermoluminescent Dosimeters (Optically Stimulated Luminescence) A TLD is exposed to ionizing radiation and excited electrons are trapped in the crystal. When the TLD is heated electrons fall back to their original state, emitting light. The light emitted is proportional to the original exposure. Lithium Fluoride is commonly used as a TLD
Film Badges	Small piece of film between metal filters. The density on the processed film is proportional to the original exposure. The metal filters allow for the estimation of the energy of radiation received. Film badges are inexpensive, easy to process, and relatively accurate but should only be worn for one month due to fogging of the film
Dosimeters	Pocket dosimeters are small ionization chambers. Dosimeters are not routinely used in the radiation therapy setting
Diodes	Small electronic probe placed on the body or inside a body cavity to measure the actual amount of radiation being delivered to a predetermined point
Geiger-Mueller Counters	Useful for locating a lost source or small amount of radioactive contamination. Limited to about 100 mrem/hour or less. With high levels of radiation, a GM counter will "swamp" causing an incorrect radiation reading
Ion Chambers	Gas filled detector used to detect or measure ionizing radiation. As ionization occurs, an electrical current is read to provide the amount of ionizing radiation. Ionization chambers are also used in the linear accelerator.
Cutie Pie Detectors	Portable ionization chamber. Useful in determining the exposure rate outside a radioactive implant patient's room
Neutron Detectors	Ionization chamber filled with BF3 gas (boron trifluoride) and is surrounded by a cadmium-loaded polyethylene sphere to slow neutrons so they can be detected efficiently

ALARA- As low as reasonably achievable

- The goal is to minimize the risk of radiation exposure and absorbed dose
- The basic methods of radiation protection are time, distance, and shielding
    - The less time you are exposed to a radiation source, the better
    - The greater distance between you and the radiation source, the better
    - The more shielding from radiation, the better. Shielding varies with varying radiation types:
        - Alpha (α) – piece of paper
        - Beta (β) - plastic, glass
        - KV Photon (x-ray) – lead
        - MV Photon – (x-ray or gamma ray) - concrete
        - Neutron (n^0) – additional shielding required due to the emission of gamma photons. Neutrons are slowed and then stopped by hydrogen rich materials such as concrete, water, or borated polyethylene combined with lead

Barrier Requirements (Shielding)

Barriers are radiation absorbing materials used to reduce radiation exposure

- Primary – materials in the radiation beam. Primary barriers are designed to attenuate the direct radiation beam
- Secondary – barriers provided in the floor, wall, and ceiling areas. Secondary barriers are designed to attenuate stray radiation

Classification of Radiation Areas (NRC Regulations CFR 10, parts 20 and 35)

- Unrestricted (uncontrolled) Area – This area may be occupied by anyone
    - A person would receive less than 2 mrem in one hour
    - No one should receive more than .1 rem in one year
- Restricted (controlled) Area – This area is occupied by radiation workers and access is controlled for the protection of individuals from exposure to radiation
    - Anyone who could receive 10% of the MPD and workers entering High and Very High Radiation Areas must be monitored
    - Approximately 50 hours/week for workers in area of 2 mrem/hour

- Radiation Area – An individual could receive a dose equivalent greater than 5 mrem in one hour at 30 cm distance from the radiation source

- High Radiation Area – An individual could receive a dose equivalent greater than .1 rem in one hour at 30 cm distance from the radiation source

- Very High Radiation Area – An individual could receive an absorbed dose greater than 500 rads in one hour at one meter from the radiation source

Required Postings of Radiation Areas

- Radiation Areas should be marked with the radiation symbol and the words **"CAUTION, RADIATION AREA"**

- High Radiation Areas should be marked with the radiation symbol and the words **"CAUTION, HIGH RADIATION AREA"** or **"DANGER, HIGH RADIATION AREA"**

- Very High Radiation Areas should be marked with the radiation symbol and the words **"GRAVE DANGER, VERY HIGH RADIATION AREA"**

- Airborne Radioactivity Areas should be marked with the radiation symbol and the words **"CAUTION, AIRBORNE RADIOACTIVITY AREA"** or **"DANGER, AIRBORNE RADIOACTIVITY AREA"**

- Rooms in which licensed material is stored should be marked with the radiation symbol and the words **"CAUTION, RADIOACTIVE MATERIALS"** or **"DANGER, RADIOACTIVE MATERIALS"**

- Containers carrying radioactive materials should be marked with the radiation symbol and the words **"CAUTION, RADIOACTIVE MATERIALS"** or **"DANGER, RADIOACTIVE MATERIALS."** The label must also provide sufficient information of the material such as: radionuclide present, estimate of the radioactivity, date that the activity is estimated, radiation levels, and kinds of materials

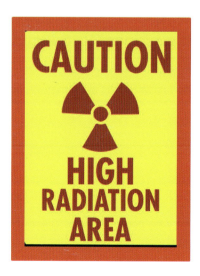

Environmental Protection

The Occupational Safety and Health Administration (OSHA) is the U.S. agency responsible for ensuring safety at work. OSHA regulates hazardous materials other than radioactive materials (e.g. processor chemicals, alcohol, germicidal cleaners, acetone, cerrobend, and batteries). Full compliance with OSHA means that any employee working with hazardous materials have "ready access" to the Materials Safety Data Sheet (MSDS)

Material Safety Data Sheet

- Sheet that lists the properties of materials that are used in the work place

- Intended to provide workers and emergency personnel procedures for handling any material or chemical in the workplace. The MSDS includes necessary information such as: melting point, boiling point, flashpoint, toxicity, health effects, first aid, reactivity, storage, disposal, protective equipment, and spill handling procedures

Toxic or Hazardous Materials

- Metals (e.g. shielding alloys)

    o Cerrobend – Hazardous due to the cadmium and lead content

        - Cadmium is a toxic metal that can cause damage to the lungs and kidneys. Cadmium can be measured in blood (recent exposure), urine (recent and past exposure), hair, or finger nails

        - Lead is a poisonous (toxic) metal that can damage the brain and other parts of the body. Lead can be measured in the blood

        - A person can become exposed to cadmium and lead by eating or drinking contaminated foods or drink. A person may also be exposed to cadmium or lead by breathing in the toxic material. Lead may also be absorbed through contact with the skin

- Chemicals (e.g. film processing)

    o Multiple Chemical Sensitivity (MCS) – chronic medical condition caused by chemical exposure

        - Chemicals involved in film processing have been linked to the cause of the newly discovered condition MCS

        - Film processing rooms should be well ventilated and the ventilation fan should be left ON at all times

- Radioactive Material (e.g. cesium, iodine)
    - The appropriate amount of shielding and labeling is required when transporting radioactive materials
    - It is important to ensure that the radiation exposure to the transporter and the general public is kept at a minimum
    - Remember: <u>Time, Distance, and Shielding</u>
    - Handling radioactive materials should be done using long-handled forceps, wearing gloves, and working behind an L block. Eating or drinking around radioactive materials is strictly prohibited. The room should have radiation monitors and the person handling the radioactive material should be wearing a personal radiation monitor such as a TLD
- Chemotherapy (containing a spill)
    - Spills involving chemotherapy materials should be handled as follows:
        - Isolate the spill and keep personnel out of the area
        - Apply double gloves, gown, and eye protection
        - When there is a threat of airborne contaminant, a National Institute for Occupational Safety and Health (NIOSH) certified respirator should be worn throughout the duration of the clean up
        - If the spill is liquid, absorb with a towel or spill kit pillow. If the spill is a solid, cover and wipe the spill with a wet absorbent gauze
        - Place all contaminated items in a biohazard bag
        - All surfaces that have been contaminated should be thoroughly cleaned with detergent and water
        - Properly dispose of all contaminated items
    - Disposal of radioactive materials can be accomplished the following ways
        - Materials with short half lives can be stored until there is sufficient radioactive decay, making the material virtually harmless
        - If the radioactive source does not exceed a certain activity limit, it can be released into the sewer system where it will decay
        - Radioactive materials can also be correctly packaged and labeled and sent away to an authorized recipient

Radiation Terms

- Exposure is a measure of the ionization produced by x-rays or gamma radiation below 3 MV
    - Roentgen (R): unit to measure radiation in air (C/kg)
- KERMA (Kinetic Energy Released in a Medium) is the sum of all initial kinetic energies from incident photons from the beam in a specified medium (air, water, phantom.) KERMA is a maximum at a surface and decreases with depth
- Absorbed Dose is a measure of the energy imparted to a mass by ionizing radiation. It can be used to prescribe patient doses in radiation therapy
    - Rad (Radiation absorbed dose)
    - Gray (Gy): 1 Gy = 100 rads
    - 1 cGy = 1 rad
- Integral Dose (volume dose) is the total energy imparted to an irradiated area by ionizing radiation (ergs/gram)
- Dose equivalent is used to equate the dose delivered by different types of radiation and their effects
    - Rem (Roentgen equivalent man) = D x Q x N
    - Sievert (Sv): 1 Sv = 100 rem
    - 1 mSv = 0.1 rem or 100 mrem
        - D = absorbed dose
        - Q = quality factor
        - N = any other factors that alter biological damage

Type of Radiation	Quality Factor (Weighting factor)
X-ray, gamma, electrons, beta	1
Neutrons	5, 10, or 20
Alpha particles	20

The quality factor takes into account the effectiveness of the **radiation** in producing biological damage

- Activity is used to describe the strength of a radioactive source based on the rate of decay. It is the number of atoms that decay per unit of time
    - Curie (Ci): 1 Ci = 3.7×10^{10} disintegrations/second
    - Becquerel (Bq): 1 Bq = 1 disintegration/second

Quality Assurance

Cobalt-60

Components

- Source is 1-2 centimeters in diameter. Because this source is not a "point source," more penumbra is present

- Housing is a lead lined steel container where the source remains in the OFF position. The source is moved to an opening in the lead shielding to the ON position. In case of fire, a failsafe device returns the source to the OFF position. The exposure rate at one meter from the source should not exceed 10 mR/hour in the OFF position

- Penumbra trimmers are collimators that can be pulled down close to the patient to reduce penumbra

How it Works

- Production of Radiation- Co-60 undergoes beta decay to Ni-60 and has two gamma emissions of 1.17 and 1.33 MeV. The beta radiation is absorbed in the cobalt and the gamma rays are used for therapy. Co-60 half life is 5.25 years and the Dmax is 0.5 centimeters

- Radiation Characteristics - The gamma rays are emitted from the nucleus of the radionuclide. These gamma rays are emitted as discrete energies

- Interaction with Matter – In soft tissue Compton scatter is the most prevalent photon interaction. Compton scatter is independent of the Z of the absorber but is dependent on the electron density. Therefore, gram for gram, bone and soft tissue absorb almost equally when undergoing Compton interactions. For this reason, bone and soft tissue do not have good contrast on MV port films

Linear Accelerators

Photon Mode:

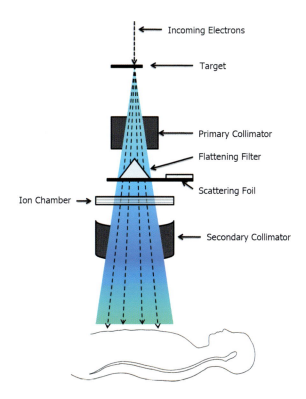

Electron Mode:

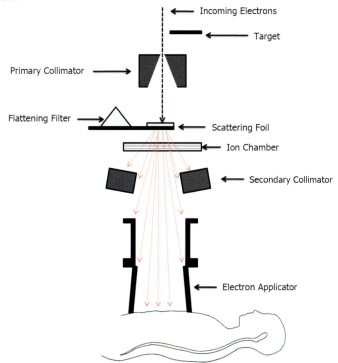

Components

- Modulator – provides electron gun and magnetron with high voltage, square, pulsed power

- Electron gun – supplies electrons needed for x-ray production and injects them into the accelerator guide

- Magnetron/Klystron – supplies RF power for the accelerator guide, pulsed simultaneously with the electron gun. Magnetrons are found in lower energy machines and produce microwaves. Klystrons are found in higher energy machines and amplify microwaves

- Waveguide – transports RF power from the magnetron to the accelerator guide. The waveguide is filled with sulphur hexafluoride (SF_6) to prevent arcing

- Circulator – one-way door in the waveguide that allows RF into the accelerator guide but not back out to prevent damage to the magnetron

- Accelerator guide – vacuum tube across which electrons are accelerated on the RF power

- Bend Magnet – forces the electrons around a bend so they exit the gantry head in the appropriate orientation for treatment

- Transmission Target – the electrons strike the target and produce x-rays. The photons exit the target in the same direction of the entering electrons

- Flattening Filter – the lead filter that attenuates some of the beam in order to provide a more uniform dose distribution

- Ion Chambers – parallel-plate chambers that check dose rate, integrated dose, and symmetry. These chambers are sealed so their response is not influenced by outside temperature and pressure

- Scattering Foil – placed in the path of the beam for electron therapy. The scattering foil spreads out the beam of electrons. When the scattering foil is in the beams path, the transmission target and flattening filter are removed

How it Works

- Production of Radiation - As the electrons are accelerated down the guide they gain energy. Then they strike a high Z target and produce x-rays via Bremsstrahlung interactions. If electron therapy is desired, the target and the flattening filter move out of the beam's path and the scattering foil moves into the beam's path

- Radiation Characteristics – The linear accelerator photon beam has a broad spectrum of energies. The maximum energy photon is the energy of the electron striking the target. The average energy is usually $1/3$ to $1/2$ the maximum energy. For electron beam mode, the following chart is useful for the estimation of electron penetration:

*E = nominal energy of the electron beam

E/2	Maximum Practical Range 2MeV/cm
E/3	80% isodose line
E/4	Therapeutic Range, 90% isodose line
E/2.33	50% isodose line

- Interaction with Matter – for low energy linacs, Compton scattering is the most prevalent interaction but as the energy increases, pair production becomes more prevalent. Pair production increases with energy above its threshold of 1.02 MV and is proportional to Z^2, so there is more absorption in bone than soft tissue with higher energy machines (>20 MV)

Superficial / Orthovoltage

Components

- Cathode Assembly - Coiled tungsten filament and negatively charged focusing cup

- Anode Assembly – The anode is positively charged and includes a tungsten target that is shielded with copper and tungsten to absorb secondary electrons and unwanted x-rays

- Tube Envelope – Houses the anode and cathode assembly in a vacuum

How it Works

- Production of Radiation – A voltage is applied between anode and cathode. Electrons are boiled off the filament in a process known as thermionic emission. The electron travels across the vacuum and hits the target producing bremmstrahlung x-rays

- Radiation Characteristics – The x-ray beam is a spectrum. Superficial units operate at 50-150 kVp and orthovoltage units operate at 150-500 kVp. Dmax is at the skin surface (no skin-sparing effect)

- Interaction with Matter – For low energy photon beams, photoelectric absorption is the most prevalent interaction. Bone absorbs more than soft tissue because its Z is higher

Machine Warm Up and Troubleshooting

Warm up

- Time Delay – real warm up that allows the filament to heat up properly. When the machine is turned on, the machine automatically goes into time delay. DO NOT BYPASS THE TIME DELAY

- Daily Check Out – verifies that the machine circuitry is functioning properly (e.g. total dose, timer, and dose rate) The operators manual gives the warm up procedure for each particular machine

Interlock Systems

- Door – the machine will not turn on if the door to the treatment room is open

Safety Lights

- Safety Lights – lights that indicate the machine is on should be located over the doors of the treatment rooms and the simulator room

Emergency Switches

- Emergency Off Buttons – these buttons are located on the control panel, in the treatment room, on the treatment table, and on the machine. These buttons are designed to disable all the control circuits and shut down the machine
- Circuit Breakers – if the emergency off button fails, the main circuit breaker is the next course of action. The circuit breaker is not normally located in the treatment room, but near the control panel. When the circuit breaker is pulled, all the power to the machine will be cut off
- Limit Switches – these limit switches are preset and prevent machine motion past the limit to prevent damage to the machine. An example of a limit switch is the gantry rotation only traveling 360° to prevent damage to the wires in the gantry

Recording Critical Machine Parameters

- Linear Accelerator – during the daily warm up the therapist will record water pressure, temperature, and fluid levels in the log book. The values should be comparable to baseline settings and previous readings. If the readings are off, notify the physicist
- Automatic Processor – the processor should be regularly checked to insure proper temperature control, adequate chemical levels, and cleanliness. A log should be kept to follow the processors performance and indications for cleaning

Associated Machine Hazards

- Electrical – linear accelerators operate at high voltages. Water can be hazardous
- Mechanical – The gantry and treatment table can cause injury by colliding
- Lasers – lasers can result in damage to the retina
- Gaseous – The treatment uses hazardous gases to operate. The machine can also create toxic fumes
    - Sulfur hexafluoride (SF^6) – colorless, odorless gas used in the treatment machine to prevent arcing in the waveguide. This gas is non-toxic but can be an asphyxiant displacing oxygen
    - Ozone – the interaction of a high energy electron beam with air can produce ozone and oxides of nitrogen. Ozone is a toxic gas that affects the respiratory system. For this reason, it is important that the treatment room be well ventilated. If the

pungent odor of the gas is detected, shut down the machine, remove the patient, and allow sufficient time for the gas to be exhausted by the normal room ventilation

Dose Verification

- Constancy of Calibration – MUST be checked weekly for linear accelerators and monthly for Cobalt – 60 units. Annual Calibrations must be performed with an ionization chamber and electrometer that have been calibrated by a NIST (National Institute of Standards and Technology) lab, and a standard phantom. Constancy checks may be performed using diodes or TLD's

- Effect of barometric pressure, temperature, and humidity on ion chambers – These chambers are not sealed and are affected by outside conditions. The chambers are calibrated by NIST labs at 22° C and 760 mm Hg pressure. All chambers must be corrected for the present conditions using the Temperature and Pressure Correction Factor:

$$CF = \frac{T + 273}{295} \times \frac{760}{P}$$

Light - Radiation Beam Coincidence

- The crosshair should represent the isocenter (axis of rotation for the collimator, gantry, and table). This can be checked using graph paper by rotating the collimator to insure that there is no "walk-out" of the crosshair. Malfunction is due to misalignment of the light field or crosshair (<2mm difference)

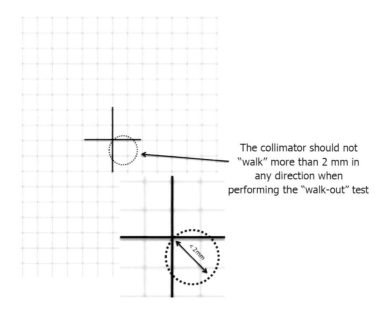

The collimator should not "walk" more than 2 mm in any direction when performing the "walk-out" test

- The light field should adequately represent the radiation field. Check this using film to insure that the field does not "walk-out" for different collimator angles. Malfunction may be due to the target, collimator, or light source. If the walk-out does not rotate, the target is causing the problem. If the walk-out does rotate, it is the collimator or light source causing the problem (<2mm difference)

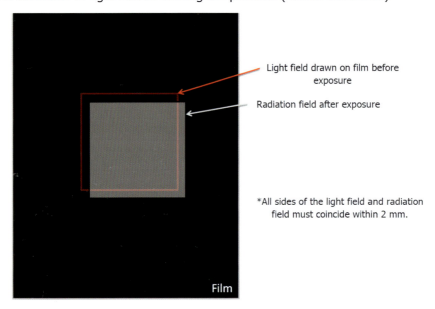

Light field drawn on film before exposure

Radiation field after exposure

*All sides of the light field and radiation field must coincide within 2 mm.

Film

- The collimator settings should agree with the measured light field. This can be checked with graph paper. Malfunction is due to the collimator drive mechanism (<2mm difference)

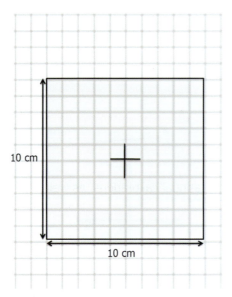

- The optical distance indicator (ODI) must be checked to insure proper representation of distances from the source/target. This is checked with the front pointer. Malfunctions include misalignment of the ODI, replacement of the light bulb, or damage to the front pointer. (< 2 mm difference)

Beam Uniformity

Check Beam Profiles for:

- Symmetry – comparison of two points equidistant from the central axis within the central 80 % of the beam ($+/-$ 2% difference)

- Flatness – variation of the beam across the central 80 % of the beam ($+/-$ 3% difference)

Rotation Check

- Clearance – to avoid mechanical collision, make sure the gantry will rotate without hitting anything (table, stretcher, IV pole etc.)

Sidelight/Laser Check

- Lateral lasers should agree with each other and the isocenter. This can be checked with the front pointer. Always check laser agreement at some point other than isocenter to insure that the lasers are not angled. Midsagittal , overhead, and backpointer lasers should also be checked. (< 2 mm difference)

Documentation of Quality Assurance Results

- By maintaining quality assurance log books, problems can be adequately followed and corrected. NRC and state regulations require that records be kept for review

Record Keeping

- Daily Checkout – if anything looks unusual or seems to be drifting out of acceptable limits, notify the physicist

- Brachytherapy Log Book – when a brachytherapy procedure is performed, all information must be recorded in a log book. This information should include: patients name, doctors signature, dates when the sources were signed out and returned, loading, number of sources, activity signed out, activity left in safe, activity returned, and the radiation safety officer on hand

- Personal Exposure Records – all films and TLD records must be kept indefinitely by the institution

- Machine Calibrations – annual calibrations, as well as the weekly/monthly checks should be kept on file. The current machine data should be kept at the console

Notification Procedures

- Treatment Machines – if something does not check out on the daily warm up, notify the physicist and do not operate the machine. If the safety lights are out, the bulb must be changed before treating. Do not operate the machine if the door interlock, timer, or other interlocks are not functioning properly

- Treatment Mistakes - if a therapist makes a mistake while delivering a patients treatment, they should notify the physician. Examples of these mistakes can be forgetting to use a wedge, not applying bolus, etc. These mistakes can alter a patients dose

- Brachytherapy Procedures – the NRC or state should be notified of the following:
    - Dose that differs from the prescribed dose by more than 10 % of the prescribed dose. This is called a recordable event
    - Dose that differs from the prescribed dose by more than 20 % of the prescribed dose. This is called a <u>misadministration</u>. Dosing the wrong patient or using a leaking source are also misadministrations

Action Plans

- Patient Movement – if the patient moves during treatment, the therapist should stop the treatment and verify the correct set up before resuming treatment. It may be necessary to set up the patient from the first step to insure proper positioning

- Mechanical Motion – if the gantry or treatment table is moving spontaneously, the therapist should press the emergency off button. If the movement is not terminated, then the circuit breaker should be used to shut down all power to the machine. Notify the physicist or engineer

- Cobalt – 60 Units – if the cobalt source does not return to its housing after the conclusion of a patients treatment, the therapist should open the door and direct the patient off of the treatment table and out of the room (if the patient is ambulatory.) If the patient is not ambulatory, the therapist should remove the patient from the table while avoiding the direct beam of the radiation source. Turn off the main switch at the control panel and notify the physicist

Radiobiology

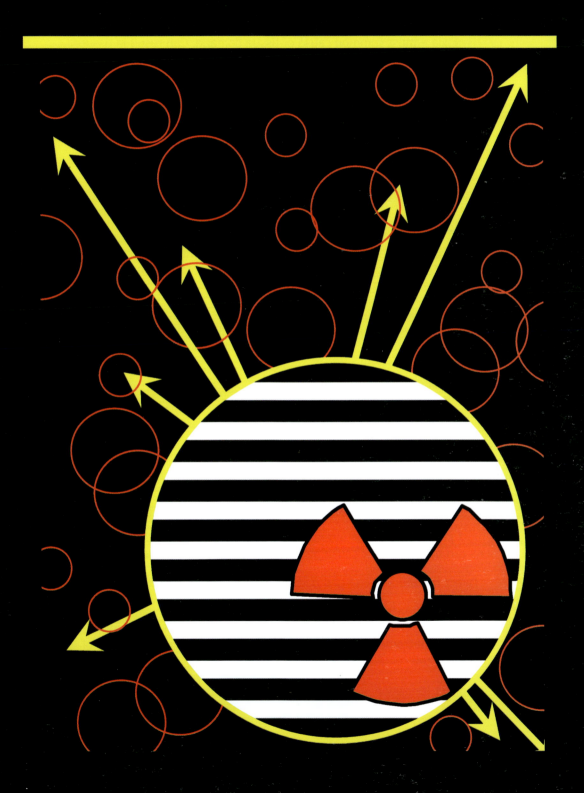

Radiobiology

- Major causes of cellular injury include:

    - Neoplasm- local invasion and destruction causes cellular inflammation or death
    - Hypoxia – most common cause of tissue damage. Can result in tissue inflammation or cell death
        - Inflammation (reversible) - local vascular dilation, cell membrane is damaged and water passes through causing redness, heat, pain, and cell swelling
    - Chemicals – cause tissue damage or cell death based on chemical interaction
    - Infection – most common cause of inflammation
    - Immunologic reactions – antigens attack the body internally or externally
    - Radiation - causes the formation of free radicals within water molecules (H- and OH-). Highly reactive free radicals can directly or indirectly destroy components of the cell

Ionizing radiation is a sufficient amount of energy transferred to a medium to cause an unstable atomic state. The atom either loses or gains an electron

- Ionizing radiation characteristics

    - Interacts and causes damage randomly
    - Energy is deposited rapidly
    - Damage cannot be distinguished from other trauma (except cataracts)
    - Changes occur after a latent period
        - Inversely related to dose administered (↑Dose = ↓Time)

- The two most probable radiation interactions are direct and indirect, and these interactions can be repaired or cause permanent damage to the cells

    - Direct Ionization – charged particles (alpha, proton, electron)
        - Interacts with the nucleus of the atom to cause damage to the DNA (target). Damage can also be done to the important macromolecules of the cell, but a "direct hit" is to the DNA of the cell
    - Indirect Ionization – x-rays, gamma rays, and neutrons
        - Indirect ionizations cause secondary effects:
            - Radiolysis – splitting of water

- An electron can be ejected to form H_2O^+. This electron can be absorbed by another atom to form H_2O^-

- These ions can form ion pairs or highly reactive free radicals. All can recombine to form water, hydrogen peroxide, or interact with the cellular components of a cell such as the nucleus

- Linear Energy Transfer (LET) – rate that energy is deposited as it travels through matter. LET varies with the speed and charge of the particle involved

  o Directly proportional to the charge

  o Inversely proportional to velocity

- Relative Biologic Effectiveness – equal doses of different LET radiations do not produce the same biologic effects

  o RBE is dependent upon radiation dose, quality, dose per fraction, number or fractions, and the type of tissue that is irradiated

$$RBE = \frac{\text{Dose from 250 KeV}}{\text{Dose of test radiation to equal same biological effect}}$$

  - If it takes 500 cGy of 250 KeV for 100% cell kill and it takes 250 cGy of neutrons for 100% cell kill, the RBE of neutrons is 2 (neutrons are 2 times more effective than 250 KeV)

Factors influencing type and extent of ionizing radiation damage

- Physical factors

  o High LET versus low LET radiation – the shoulder region of the cell survival curve is decreased or absent when high LET radiation is utilized. This results in a steeper curve

  o More damage is done with high LET in a shorter path of travel than low LET. The biological effect of high LET radiation is greater than low LET radiation because high LET radiation deposits all of its energy inside the cell causing significant damage to the DNA. Low LET radiation causes less serious DNA breaks than can easily be repaired

  o Low dose rates are less efficient in producing cell damage than high dose rates. Cells can repair damage with low enough dose rates

- The cell survival curve is a semi log graph that depicts the number of cells surviving versus the radiation dose delivered. For photons, the curve has an initial shoulder, and then the slope changes. The shoulder of the curve corresponds to single event killing and the amount of sub lethal damage repaired
    - D_q - measure of the width of the shoulder of the curve. It signifies a build up or accumulation of damage before cell death actually occurs. It is called the quasi-threshold dose because there is no true threshold dose
    - D_o - the final slope of the curve. As the dose increases the curve straightens to a line of constant slope, reflecting a direct logarithmic dose-response relationship. This is the dose required to reduce the surviving fraction to 37% of its previous value (cell kill). May be called D_{37}
    - n – number obtained by extrapolation backwards from the final slope of the curve to where is crosses the Y axis. This signifies the number of targets hit

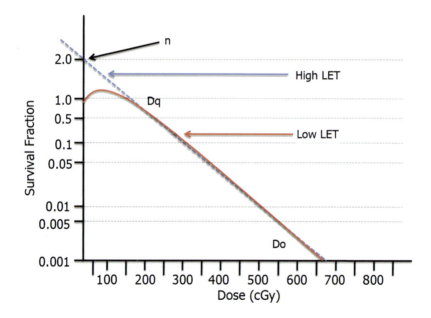

- When photons are delivered in a fractionated schedule (daily treatments), the shoulder may appear multiple times because of cellular repair between treatments.

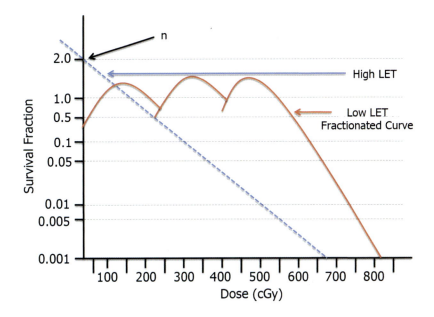

- The cell survival curve is a straight line for densely ionizing, high LET radiations (e.g. protons)

- Proton depth dose curves have a sudden deposit of energy resulting in a peak of the curve. This peak is known as Bragg peak

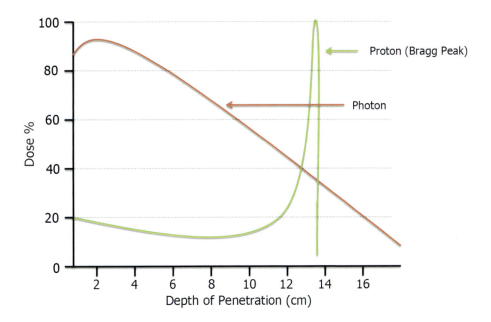

- The therapeutic ratio is the ratio of the ability to control a tumor versus the amount of complications or severity with that dose regimen. The larger the difference (or therapeutic ratio), the greater the effectiveness of that treatment

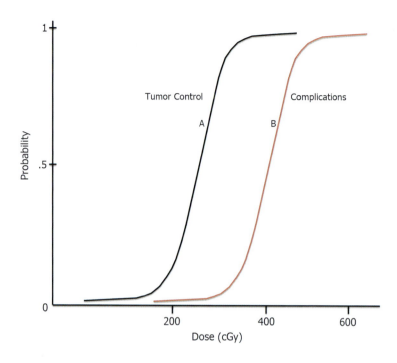

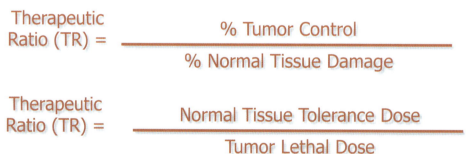

- Chemical factors
    - The most potent chemical factor in ionizing radiation is the presence of oxygen. The oxygen fixation hypothesis states that oxygen may enhance the formation of free radicals and make these damages permanent by preventing the repair of damaged cells
        - Most significant with low LET radiations where indirect interactions predominate
        - As the availability of O_2 decreases, cell response decreases

- Oxygen Enhancement Ratio (OER) – compares the response of the cells to radiation with and without the presence of oxygen

$$OER = \frac{\text{Anoxic radiation dose}}{\text{Dose in oxic conditions to produce same effect}}$$

- If D_0 is 300 cGy under hypoxic conditions, and is reduced to 100 cGy under oxic conditions, the OER is 3.0
- For mammalian cells, the OER for x-rays is usually 2.5 – 3.0. (In anoxic conditions, the dose of radiation needs to be 2.5 – 3.0 times greater than the dose in oxic conditions)
- OER is less significant for neutrons (1.6) and is negligible for high LET radiations (1.0)

- Biological factors

  Phases of the cell cycle

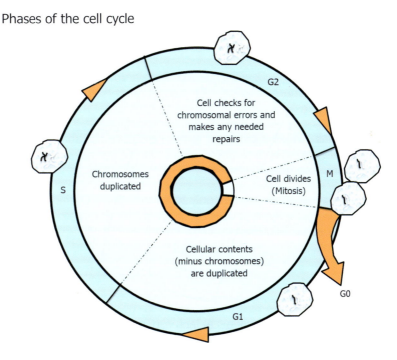

- M (Mitosis) – cell division

- G1 – gap between mitosis and DNA synthesis, rapid growth and active metabolism – RNA synthesis, in late G1 cells commit to replication

- G0 – resting phase, fully functioning, point of decision to replicate

- S – DNA synthesis (replication)

- G2 – gap between DNA synthesis and mitosis, cell prepares for division

Cells are most sensitive to radiation during the M phase of the cell cycle and least sensitive to radiation during the S phase

- Cells have the ability to repair sublethal damage. Cell survival increases if the radiation dose is administered in fractions as opposed to a single dose to the same total dose
    - Hyperfractionation – treating more than once a day, usually twice a day. Approximately 6 hours should elapse between the first and second treatment of the day
    - Hypofractionation – treating less than once a day. Fewer treatments with higher doses. Hypofractionation can also be single high doses for 2 to 3 treatments spaced about a week apart
    - Accelerated radiotherapy – the overall therapy time is shortened. There are usually two treatments a day, and the dose per fraction may be slightly reduced.
- The biological effect of radiation on cells is dependent upon the 4 R's:
    - **R**epopulation - Both normal tissues and tumor cells may divide between fractions. Radiation is more effective when the tumor cells are more actively mitotic than the normal tissue
    - **R**edistribution (reassortment) - Both normal tissue and tumor cells can move to more resistant (S phase) or more sensitive (M phase) within the cell cycle
    - **R**epair - Normal cells and tumor cells have the ability to repair sublethal damage. When well oxygenated, mature normal cells repair better than immature tumor cells
    - **R**eoxygenation (applies only to tumor cells) - During fractionated treatments, hypoxic cells can gain access to oxygen and become more radiosensitive. When some of the tumor cells are killed, the more hypoxic cells become better oxygenated

Radiosensitivity

- Ionizing radiation is more effective against cells that are actively mitotic, undifferentiated (immature, stem, or precursor), and have a long dividing future. (Law of Bergonie and Tribondeau, 1906)
- Radiosensitivity of an organ is a function of the most sensitive cell that it contains
    - Parenchyma – cells that make up the organ
    - Stroma – supporting vasculature of the organ

        Example: The parenchyma of the liver is radioresistant while its supporting vasculature (stroma) is more radiosensitive, making the liver a radiosensitive structure

Cellular Response

- Cellular response to radiation treatment is a function of:
    - Dose administered
    - Volume Irradiated
    - Time of observation after irradiation
- Response manifests as either early (acute) or late (chronic)
    - Late changes are early changes that were irreversible and progressive. The latent period of these changes is inversely proportional to the radiation dose
    - The damage done can have somatic or genetic effects on the cells of the body
        - Somatic – cells of the body
            - Can cause non-specific radiation induced "life shortening"
            - Decrease the number of parenchymal cells and blood vessels
            - Cellular response to radiation can be seen as:
                - Division delay – the mitotic index is disrupted and this causes fewer cells to divide
                - Interphase death – most cells require a higher dose to kill post mitotic cells (except lymphocytes, only 50 cGy can cause interphase death)
                - Reproductive failure/mitotic death – chromosomal damage inhibits cell production. This is the most common cause of cell death
                - Apoptosis – natural programmed cell death
        - Genetic – reproductive cells (germ cells)
            - Homeostasis is the maintaining of normal cellular function and can be disrupted by radiation, causing breaks in genetic material resulting in:
                - Restitution – Single radiation induced break resulting in two fragments. Fragments can rejoin resulting in no damage

- Structural changes – these damaged cells can survive, resulting in the inability to reproduce, or the ability to continue the production of more damaged cells

- Gene amplification – DNA replication becomes selective and reproduces a certain gene at an increased rate.

- Chromosome translocation – broken cell fragments try to repair and rejoin

- Gene transposition – cells create the wrong genetic codes

- Mutation – missing an element

Patient Care

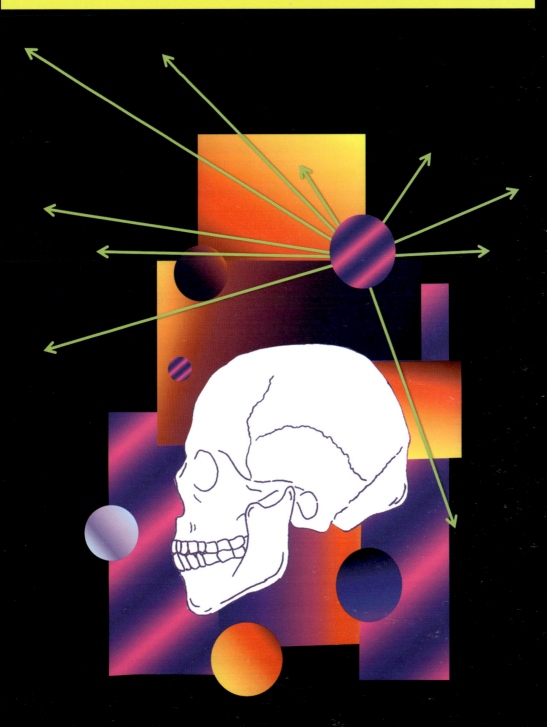

Ethical and Legal Aspects

- Patient's Rights
    - Informed consent – patient must be informed of
        - Nature of procedure, treatment, or disease
        - Expectations of treatment and likelihood of success
        - Treatment alternatives and outcome without treatment
        - Known risk factors of treatment
    - Confidentiality
        - HIPAA (Health Insurance Portability and Accountability Act) – provides federal protection for personal health information, and gives the patient rights to that information
        - Patient information must be kept in a secure area, not be revealed without proper consent, and can only be discussed with those directly involved in treatment. The exception is if the life of the patient or safety of a third party is jeopardized
    - Additional Rights
        - Patient's Bill of Rights - Implies a patient's legal right to affect treatment outcome through the use of:
            - Do Not Resuscitate (DNR) orders – part of the Public Health Law that allows the legal avenue to withhold cardiopulmonary resuscitation
            - Living Will – legal document in which patients have control of their future, and the family's wishes do not override the patient's. Living wills relieve doctors and hospitals of legal responsibility. A signature must be witnessed by two disinterested individuals that are not related to the patient, are not mentioned in the will, and have no claim to the estate
            - Health Care Proxies (substitute) – legal document that gives a family member or friend (referred to as the health care provider) the authority to make critical decisions if the patient becomes incapacitated
            - Research Participation – patient has the right to refuse to participate in research, and has rights to receiving full explanation of research. A consent form must be signed to participate, but the patient can withdraw from research at any time. The doctor can stop a patient's treatment at any time if the patient is not responding well to treatment

- Legal Issues
    - Civil Law – non-criminal disputes such as disagreements over contracts, property ownership, and personal property damages
    - Tort Law – a legal wrong against a person or property, excluding contract disagreements or disputes
        - Intentional tort
            - Civil assault - threat of touching in an injurious way. This can be avoided by explaining the full procedure to the patient beforehand
            - Civil battery – touching without permission
            - False imprisonment – intentional confinement (such as immobilization devices)
            - Libel – written defamation of character (everything in a patient's chart is subject to review)
            - Slander – oral defamation of character
            - Invasion of privacy – information released, or patient exposed improperly or unnecessarily
        - Unintentional tort
            - Negligence – neglect or omission of reasonable care
            - Malpractice - result of professional misconduct, incompetence, or lack of skills
    - Scope of practice for a profession – written context of what the professional can do based on education and preparation
    - Standard of practice for a profession – delineates the proper procedure and how an action should be performed
    - Personal liability – must take responsibility of own actions
    - Doctrine of respondent superior – holding the employer responsible for negligent acts of an employee
    - Res Ipsa Loquitor ("the thing speaks for itself") – a defendant can explain events and a court can decide outcome with no witness present
    - Doctrine of forseeability - knowledge of actions or lack of information that could cause injury
    - Risk management – identifies causes of accidents and implements programs to prevent them

- Incident reports – report of any happening that is not routine operation. The report should not contain opinions, accusation, or conjecture, only the facts

- Good Samaritan laws – laws that exist in most states to limit the legal liability of health care professionals who help in an emergency situation outside the work setting

Interpersonal Communication

- Modes of communication

  - Verbal communication – includes spoken and written words

  - Nonverbal communication – includes gestures and actions. Physical appearance, facial expressions, eye contact, and touch form the basis of nonverbal communication

- Challenges in communication

  - Patient Characteristics

    - Cultural diversity – one generation passing specific behaviors and characteristics to the next

    - Emotional status – patient and family members in the grieving process may block effective communication

      – Grieving process: denial, anger, bargaining, depression, and acceptance

    - Physical or sensory impairments – Americans with Disabilities Act 1990 (ADA) provides civil rights protection to those with disabilities

    - Physical impairment – any physiological disorder or condition including cosmetic disfigurement

    - Mental impairment – mental retardation, organic brain syndrome, emotional and mental illness, and specific learning disabilities

  - Patient Support

    - Hospice – palliative care for terminally ill patients. Requirements for hospice care include: terminal illness, life expectancy of less than six months, and care within a defined geographic location

Pain Assessment and Management

- Generalized side effects and medications
    - Antiemetic (nausea) - Torecan, Norazine, Compazine
    - Analgesic (pain killer) - Tylenol, Percocet, MS Contin
    - Anti-Inflammatory - Hydrocortisone, Diprolene
    - Anti-Diarrheal- Imodium, Lomotil
    - Protectant- Carafate (adheres to ulcer site; inhibits pepsin)
    - Topical or Oral Anesthetic- Xylocaine elixir
    - Anti-microbial (kills or inhibits growth of microorganisms) - Peridex
- Skin reactions (specific to area in treatment port)
    - Stage 1 Inflammation – color pinkish red, slight edema
    - Stage 2 Inflammation and dry desquamation – skin becomes dry and scaly due to shedding of the epidermis, this is usually itchy
    - Stage 3 Inflammation, edema, and moist desquamation – skin thins and starts to weep because the epithelial layer has lost its integrity. Treatment may be temporarily discontinued to allow skin cells to repair and heal
    - Stage 4 Depilation of the hair in the treatment field – permanent hair loss
    - Late side effects (6 months to 5 years after treatment)
        - Fibrosis – tissue scarring
        - Telangiectasis – abnormal dilation of superficial capillaries and arteries
        - Impairment of lymphatic drainage (lymphedema)
    - Management
        - Cleanse skin with mild soap, dry skin well (especially in skin folds), and use cornstarch to reduce moisture
        - Avoid tight fitting clothes and harsh fabrics
        - Avoid exposing skin in the treatment field to extreme hot or cold temperature, direct sunlight, chemicals (deodorants, chlorine)

- Anorexia – loss of appetite resulting in weight loss. Major contributor of cachexia, or a physical wasting with loss of weight and muscle mass caused by disease
    - Causes – disease process, side effect of cancer therapy, stress, anxiety, depression, alteration in normal life style, fatigue, taste alterations, pain, and infection
    - Management
        - Encourage patients to eat frequently (many small meals) and avoid drinking while eating
        - Encourage nutritional supplements, and high protein, high caloric foods
        - Exercise prior to meals and rest when fatigued
        - Take analgesics before eating if pain is present
- Fatigue
    - Causes – release of waste into the blood stream as a result of cell destruction. Increase in basal metabolic rate (calories burned) resulting in increased energy consumption. Increase in anabolic cellular proliferation (cell production) and differentiation (needed for normal tissue cellular repair in the treatment field)
    - Management
        - Assess duration, intensity and time when fatigue is greatest/least
        - Encourage patient to rest when fatigued
        - Force fluids
        - Encourage patients to pace themselves and allow for plenty of rest time
- Bone marrow depression – not usually a problem unless 25% or more of active bone marrow is in the treatment field
    - Bone marrow production

Site	Approximate %
Skull	10%
Ribs/Sternum	20%
Pelvic Bones	30%
Vertebrae	25%
Scapula	10%
Femur/Humerus	5%

- Management

    - Assess the situation looking for problems associated with infection, anemia, neutropenia, and bleeding

Site Specific Side Effects

Scalp

- Alopecia – extent of hair lost is dependent upon treatment field and dose

    - Temporary hair loss – 1500 – 3000 cGy
    - Hair loss varies with patient – 3000 – 4500 cGy
    - Permanent hair loss – 4500 cGy and up
    - Management

        - Minimize hair loss by using a mild shampoo and a soft brush with wide teeth
        - Avoid sun exposure, hot rollers, hair dryers, hair sprays, and perms
        - Encourage patient to purchase a wig prior to complete hair loss

- Edema – inflammatory reaction resulting in swelling

    - Signs of increased intracranial pressure include: change in mental status, confusion, hypertension, decrease in pulse and respiration, headaches, nausea, motor and sensory changes, and vomiting
    - Management

        - Corticosteroids are prescribed during brain irradiation to prevent or reduce swelling

Head and Neck

- Xerostomia – dryness of the mucous membranes in the oral cavity

    - Causes include radiation therapy, tumors involving the salivary glands, and some medications
    - Management

        - Oral lubricants (artificial saliva), minimize dental caries (cavities), consistent mouth care, and avoid nicotine, alcohol, and irritating foods

- Taste Alterations
  - Causes
    - Taste bud destruction due to radiation therapy
    - Reduction in saliva
    - Waste products of cellular destruction and disease process (cancer cells release bi-products that cause a bitter taste)
  - Management
    - Maintain hydration of mucous membranes (use artificial saliva)
- Mucositis/Stomotitis – inflammation of the mucosal surfaces
  - Most common oral infections
    - Candidiasis (thrush) – white patches on tongue and oral mucosa
    - Herpes simplex – common viral infection (painful vesicles on lips that rupture and become encrusted)
    - Gram negative bacteria – raised, painful, shiny, reddened base anywhere in the mouth
  - Management
    - Daily oral assessments
    - Decrease trauma to mucosa, avoid alcohol and tobacco
    - Increase protein, calorie, and fluid intake with meals (avoid spices, and hot foods)
    - Oral hygiene regimen (use soft bristle tooth brush)
    - Medications: Viscous Xylocaine, Peridex, Nizoral, Diflucan, Analgesics
- Pharyngitis/Esophagitis - inflammation of esophagus or pharynx resulting in dysphagia; may require treatment break if severe
  - Management
    - Increase protein and calorie intake with meals, choose soft foods with smooth textures
    - Take analgesics and/or protectants prior to eating to limit discomfort
    - Medications: Carafate, Xylocaine, Analgesics

- Ear Pain

    - Caused by inner, middle, or outer ear being treated with radiation therapy. Pain from edema

    - Management

        - Anesthetic ear drops

- Late Head and Neck Side Effects

    - Atrophy of skin – 4-6 weeks after treatment is completed

    - Lenticular opacities – if the eye is in the treatment field, 300 – 1000 cGy

    - Cataracts – 1000 cGy total, or 200 cGy single treatment

    - Fistulas and Ulcerations – due to decreased vascularity

    - Osteoradionecrosis – usually in the mandible, tooth decay and infections can lead to necrosis of the bone (alcohol and tobacco intake increase likelihood)

Chest/Upper Back

- Esophagitis – indigestion, nausea and vomiting

    - Causes

        - Epithelial cells lining the esophagus, stomach, or intestines are destroyed producing toxic waste products that cause nausea

    - Management

        - Assessment of frequency, duration, circumstances, patterns etc.

        - Provide and encourage hydration

        - Antiemetics for nausea

        - Use relaxation and distraction techniques

        - Pay close attention to lab work (electrolyte levels)

- Pneumonitis

    - Caused by the destruction of cells lining the alveoli causing inflammation and fluid accumulation. Factors are dose and lung volume irradiated

        - 25% or less – asymptomatic

        - Greater than 25% - cough, dyspnea, fever, weakness

        - 75% or more – irreversible damage

- Management
  - Steroids and antibiotics to prevent infection

Abdomen/Lower Back

- Nausea/Vomiting – cause and management the same as with chest and upper back
- Diarrhea
  - Caused by radiation destruction of highly proliferative epithelial cells lining the intestines
  - Management
    - Assessment of onset, duration, character, amount, and frequency
    - Promote hydration
    - Assessment of skin integrity of perianal area
    - Stress the importance of skin care (baths, ointment use)
    - Avoid foods that are fibrous, greasy, or spicy. Avoid milk products
    - Medications: Anti-diarrheal- Lomotil, Imodium
- Cystitis – inflammation of the lining of the bladder. May present with urgency, frequency, burning, lower back pain, and blood in urine
  - Management
    - Assessment of onset, duration, frequency, and characteristics of urine
    - Assess for signs: elevated temperature, pus in urine, foul smelling urine
    - Increase fluid intake to at least 3000 ml/day
    - Maintain urine pH of 7.0 or less (suggest ascorbic acid or cranberry juice)
    - Medications: Antibiotics, Anesthetics (Urised, Pyridium)
- Sexual dysfunction
  - Occurs when testes or ovaries are located in the treatment field. Developing sperm and ova are very radiosensitive. The amount of dysfunction is dependent upon dose, fractionation, volume of tissue treated, and physiological and psychological status of the patient

- Male – effect of radiation on testes
  - < 500 cGy (temporary sterility)
  - > 500 cGy (permanent sterility)
- Management
  - Emotional support. Suggest counseling and encourage patient to express feelings and concerns
- Female – when ovaries are in the treatment field, the patient may experience:
  - Temporary or permanent sterility (dose and age related)
  - Decreased libido
  - Chromosomal damage
  - Atrophy of vaginal mucosa, shrinkage of vaginal size, decrease in vaginal lubrication
  - Inflammation of the mucous membranes in the vagina causing ulceration and edema
- Female – when the vagina is located in the treatment field
  - Stenosis, fibrosis, decreased lubrication, disruption of epithelial integrity, decreased libido
- Management
  - Dilator use (instruct patient)
  - Utilize water based lubricant (KY)
  - Avoid sexual intercourse when mucositis is present
  - Prevent infection
  - Emotional support

Blood Studies

- Creatinine blood tests – evaluates kidney function. This is important to assess prior to injecting contrast media to visualize the kidneys

- Hemoglobin (Hb) – chemical compound in red blood cells that carries oxygen. Should maintain hemoglobin level >10 g/dl. Low LET radiation will have greater effects due to OER (Oxygen Enhancement Ratio)

    o Normal values

        ▪ Men - 15.5 g/dl

        ▪ Women – 13.7 g/dl

        ▪ Average – 12-16 g/dl

- White Blood Cell count (WBC) – fight infection. Important to assess the Absolute Neutrophil Count (ANC). A low neutrophil count makes a person more vulnerable to infection

    o WBC Normal range - 4,500-10,000 white blood cells per microliter (mcL)

- Platelets – main function is to aid in coagulation

    o Normal range – 150,000 – 400,000 per microliter (dangerous if count decreases below 50,000 during treatment)

Physical Assistance and Transfer

- Good body mechanics include balance, alignment, and proper movement

    o Balance – have a strong base of support, spread feet apart so the body is balanced while standing

    o Alignment (posture) – when lifting, keep back straight, bend knees, and avoid twisting. Keep object close to the body and balanced over both feet

    o Proper movement – when lifting, use abdominal and leg muscles rather than back muscles. Bend knees and lift with legs

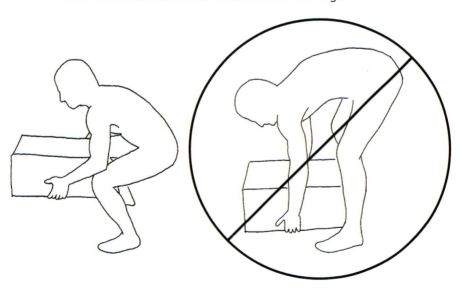

- Positioning and Monitoring of Accessory Medical Equipment
    - Intravascular catheters
        - Assessment – signs of infiltration (redness, swelling, tenderness, heat)
        - Position patient to promote patency (open flow)
    - Chest tubes
        - Assessment – ensure properly functioning system, no bubbling in water seal bottle (bubbling suggests a leak), check for air leaks in system, tube should be securely placed
        - Tachypnea (fast breathing), tachycardia (fast heart rate), anxiety, and restlessness are indicators of increased air in the pleural space
        - Infection – high WBC, increased temperature, purulent drainage
        - Cautions - Maintain sterility and patency; if tube becomes dislodged or bottle breaks, then apply clamps as near to the patient as possible; if tube displaced from chest, then have patient exhale forcefully (cover chest wall with petroleum gauze)
    - Oxygen therapy – the goal is to supply a sufficient amount of O_2 to the tissues until normal metabolic needs are met
        - Low flow systems – nasal cannula, simple O_2 mask
        - High flow systems – venturi mask
        - Assess patency (ensure the system is delivering the prescribed amount of O_2), patient's respiratory status, vital signs, anxiety, hydration, blood gases etc.
        - Management
            - No smoking around O_2 administration (extremely flammable)
            - Oxygen cylinders must be secured when stored or in use
            - O_2 administration requires a doctor's order

- Nasogastric (NG) tube
  - Management
    - Carefully transfer patient, being careful not to dislodge or place tension on tube
    - Assess patient for complications including pulmonary aspiration of formula or diarrhea. Notify doctor for any of the above
- Urinary Catheter – two commonly used types:
  - Straight or single lumen
  - Foley, retention double or triple lumen
  - Management
    - Encourage patient to drink plenty of fluids
    - Be aware of color, clarity, and overall appearance of urine and report any abnormality to the physician
    - Avoid yanking, pulling, or kinking of tube (clamp should be open)
    - Report any complaints of urgency, hesitancy, or dysuria to the physician
- Tracheostomy tube
  - Endotracheal tube – tube passed via the nose or mouth, through the larynx, and into the trachea as a means of providing an airway
  - Tracheostomy tube – artificial hole made in the trachea into which a tube is placed
  - Usage
    - To establish and maintain a patient's airway
    - To prevent aspiration by sealing off the trachea from the digestive tract (in unconscious or paralyzed patient)
    - To permit removal of tracheobronchial secretions in patients who can't cough adequately
    - To ventilate patient that can't be ventilated by face mask

- Management

    - Maintain patient airway, any distress merits a call to nurse or physician

    - Assess the patient's respiratory status to determine if suctioning is necessary; when respirations are noisy, pulse and respiratory rates are increased, the patient needs to be suctioned

    - Encourage patients to use a humidifier to moisten tenacious secretions

    - Assist the patient in alternative modes of communication

    - Provide emotional support

- Pacemaker – treatment for cardiac arrhythmias

    - Usage

        - Provides an artificial pacing mechanism that delivers stimulus to the heart

    - Management

        - If the pacemaker is in the treatment field, the manufacturer should be contacted to verify that treatment to the pacemaker will not cause malfunction. The following information should be available:

            - Type of pacemaker
            - Rate
            - Milliamperage
            - Manufacturer
            - Model number

        - Be alert to signs that may require physician attention such as: pain, tenderness at point of insertion, fever, pulse rate above or below average

        - Most manufacturers have not done research on doses greater than 500 cGy. Blocking the pacemaker should be a routine safety measure unless larger dose tolerances can be documented

Medical Emergencies

- Allergic reactions (latex, contrast, tape)
    - Signs are nausea, vomiting, itching, fainting, pain, edema, convulsions, cardiac arrhythmias
- Cardiac Arrest
    - Signs are clutching at chest, sweating, pallor, shortness of breath (SOB), irregular heartbeat
    - Management
        - Stop all physical activity and lie or sit down
        - Initiate Cardiopulmonary Resuscitation (CPR) and direct current shock (defibrillation)
        - Chew an aspirin to dissolve clot following cardiac arrest
- Other medical disorders
    - Partial Seizure - Usually begins in the hand or foot and moves up the extremity. Patient appears alert, but is nonresponsive
    - Petit Mal Seizure - Occurs without warning and is more common during childhood and adolescence. Patient abruptly stops all activity and may exhibit eye or muscle fluttering
    - Grand Mal Seizure - Seizure is typically preceded by symptoms such as certain smells, flashing lights, spots before the eyes, dizziness that serve as warnings of impending seizures. Patient generally loses consciousness
    - Management
        - Place patient on the ground or floor in a safe area, preferably on their right side. Remove any nearby objects. Loosen any clothing around the head or neck. **Do not** try to wedge the mouth open or place an object between the teeth, and **do not** attempt to restrain movements
- Diabetic reactions
    - Hyperglycemia (elevated blood glucose levels)
        - Signs and symptoms include: nausea, vomiting, polyuria (excessive urination), polydipsia (patient takes in excessive amounts of water), headaches, hot, dry, and flushed skin, increased thirst, weakness, drowsiness, altered mental state, inability to speak, or paralysis

- Management
    - Requires intravenous fluids and may require insulin. Deadly if left untreated
- Hypoglycemia (low blood glucose levels) – results from insulin overdose, inadequate food intake, increased exercise, nutritional and fluid imbalances
    - Signs and symptoms include: excessive sweating, feeling faint, cool, moist, and pale skin, confusion or behavior changes, difficulty talking, complaints of feeling weak or shaky, blurred or double vision, and increased heart rate. (usually a sudden onset)
    - Management
        - Mild cases can be treated quickly by eating or drinking a small amount of glucose rich food. If left untreated, hypoglycemia can cause confusion, clumsiness, or fainting. Severe hypoglycemia can lead to seizures, coma, and even death

Infection Control

- Terminology and Basic concepts
    - Asepsis – free from all disease causing contaminants (e.g. bacteria, fungi, viruses, and parasites)
    - Nosocomial infections – infections that develop in the hospital or are acquired in the hospital
    - Universal precautions
        - Blood and body fluid precautions apply to all patients (universal), and should be treated as if known to be infectious for HIV, HBV, and other blood borne pathogens
        - Universal precautions address the prevention of needle sticks and the use of protective equipment such as: gloves, gowns, masks, and eye protection
            - OSHA (Occupational Safety and Health Administration) adopted the universal precautions concept and requires that medical facilities provide occupational exposure training and offer the hepatitis B vaccine at no cost to the health care worker
        - Body substance isolation – requires the isolation of all bodily fluids for all patients (through the use of gloves or other protective gear)

- Strict Isolation

    - Prevents the transmission of infections through direct contact or air

    - A private room with the door closed and negative air flow (special ventilation) is required

    - Anyone entering the room should wear gown, gloves and a mask

    - Hand washing is required after exiting the room. Contaminated articles should be discarded or bagged and labeled to be sent away for decontamination

- Contact Isolation

    - Prevents the transmission of diseases that are spread by close or direct contact

    - A private room is required

    - Masks, gown, and gloves should be worn if close contact takes place

    - Hand washing is required after exiting the room; contaminated articles should be discarded or bagged and labeled to be sent for decontamination

- Respiratory Isolation

    - Prevents the transmission of large droplets of infectious pathogens over a short distance

    - A private room is required

    - Masks are needed if close contact occurs (gowns and gloves are not necessary)

    - Hand washing is required after exiting the room; contaminated articles should be discarded or bagged and labeled to be sent for decontamination

- Tuberculosis (TB)/Acid-fast Bacilli (AFB) Isolation

    - Prevents the airborne transmission of active TB

    - A private room with the door closed and negative air flow (special ventilation) is required

    - Surgical masks are not effective, thus a particular respirator is recommended (gowns and gloves are not necessary)

- Hand washing is required after exiting the room; contaminated articles should be discarded or bagged and labeled to be sent for decontamination

- Enteric Precautions

  - Prevents transmission of infections by direct or indirect contact with fecal material

  - A private room is not necessary

  - Masks are not necessary and gowns are not needed unless there is risk of contact with fecal material (gloves are needed for touching potentially infected materials)

  - Hand washing is required after exiting the room; contaminated articles should be discarded or bagged and labeled to be sent for decontamination

- Drainage and Secretion Precautions

  - Prevents transmission of infections by direct or indirect contact with secretions or drainage from an infected body site

  - A private room is not necessary

  - Masks are not necessary and gowns are not needed unless there is risk of contact with infectious material (gloves are needed for touching potentially infected materials)

  - Hand washing is required after exiting the room; contaminated articles should be discarded or bagged and labeled to be sent for decontamination

o Hand washing is the most important way to prevent spread of infection

- Personnel

  - Hand washing between all patient's

  - Wear clothing that is washable and easily cleaned

  - Keep work area, floors, tables, and working surfaces clean

  - When possible encourage patients to change clothes in cubicle

  - A major source of bacteria in the air is soiled linen and clothes

  - Follow strict protocol for procedures that require sterile technique (suctioning, catherization, dressing changes, etc.)

- Sterile Technique - process which destroys all microbial life forms, including resistant spores
    - Clean according to manufacturer's recommendations
        - Methods: Autoclave (heat, steam, and pressure), Gas sterilization, Chemical sterilization (Amphyl, Cidex)
- Disinfection - process which reduces microbial life forms and can range from high level disinfection to low level disinfection. Low level disinfection is also called sanitization
    - Methods: very hot to boiling water, liquid chemicals, chlorine compounds
- Antiseptic - agent that will prevent the growth or arrest the development of microorganisms

- Cycle of Infection
    - Causative Agent (Source) - Bacteria, virus, fungi
    - Reservoir (for microorganism growth) - Animate or inanimate
    - Portal of Exit - Respiratory tract, GI tract, GU Tract, skin, transplacental
    - Mode of Transmission - Contact (direct or indirect), droplet, airborne, vector
    - Portal of Entry - Respiratory tract, GI tract, GU tract, skin
    - Susceptible Host - Age, immunologic status, radiation therapy, intrusive procedures, malnutrition

- Method of Transmission
    - Contact - most frequent spread for nosocominal
        - Direct (physical transfer) - caregiver physically touches infected patient or bodily fluids
        - Indirect - needle stick, bedpan, intravenous catheter
    - Droplet - heavy particles do not linger in air very long. Three feet or less for exposure. Usually spread by coughing and sneezing (chicken pox, TB)
    - Airborne - through air over long distance. Six feet or more for exposure. Agents can linger in air for a few days
    - Common Inanimate Vehicles – formite is a contaminated, inanimate object such as food, water, blood, feces (Hepatitis A, Polio)
    - Vector Borne - disease carrying insect or animal. Transfers infectious agent to host (mosquito, ticks)

Chemotherapeutic Drugs

Administration

- Intravenous – a majority of chemotherapeutic drugs are administered intravenously. For extended treatments, catheters can be placed in the patient's vessels to maintain an access point and avoid repeated needle sticks. The common systems are Hickman line, Port-A-Cath, and PICC line

Side Effects

- Chemotherapeutic drugs have a greater effect on rapidly dividing cells. This applies to both tumor cells and normal cells, such as blood cells and the cells lining the mouth, stomach, and intestines. Common side effects include:

    - Myleosuppression – decrease in white blood cells, red blood cells, and platelets, leading to infections, anemia, and bleeding
    - Nausea
    - Vomiting
    - Hair loss
    - Infertility

- Treatment

    - Allogenic or autologous bone marrow transplants may be necessary if patient becomes too immunosuppressed
        - Allogenic – bone marrow cells are taken from a donor
        - Autologous – bone marrow cells are removed from the patient before treatment, multiplied, and re-injected

- Chemotherapeutic agents are associated with organ specific toxicities. Examples include:

    - Doxorubicin (adriamyicin) – cardiotoxicity
    - Bleomycin – interstitial lung disease
    - MOPP therapy for Hodgkin disease – secondary neoplasms

Treatment Planning and Delivery

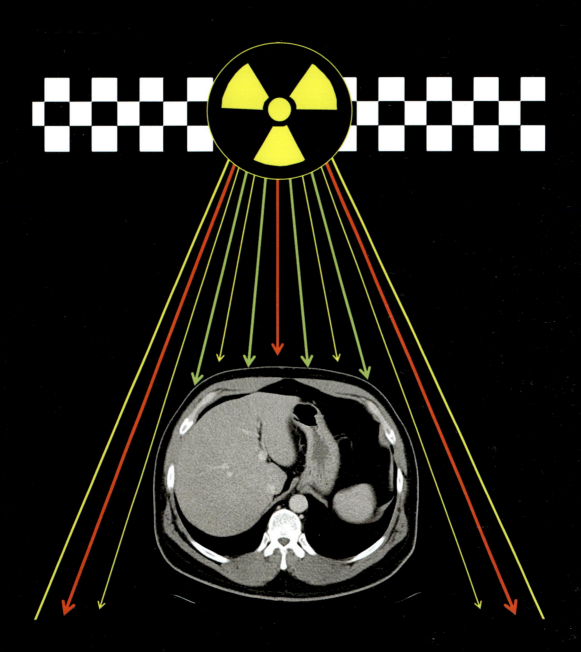

Digital Imaging

Terminology

- Pixel - a two dimensional unit based on the matrix size and the field of view. The basic picture element to make a 2 dimensional image

- Voxel - a three dimensional unit that includes slice thickness. A three dimensional representation that is short for "volume pixel" (the smallest distinguishable box)

- Matrix - an array of numbers in rows and columns. The horizontal lines in matrices are called rows and the vertical lines are called columns. Determines the scan resolution. The higher the matrix, the better the resolution. Reconstruction takes longer with higher resolution and patient exposure may be greater

- Field of View (FOV) - the maximum diameter of the area of the scan that can be seen in the reconstructed image

- Digitally Reconstructed Radiograph (DRR) - computer generated two dimensional radiograph displaying skeletal anatomy rendered from a three dimensional data set, such as CT or MRI

- Beam's Eye View (BEV) - viewpoint of the radiation beam as it travels from the radiation source

- Image Registration - the process of spatially aligning two or more image datasets (e.g., CT, MR, PET, contrast and non-contrast studies) of the same area, taken at different times

- Image Fusion - combining image datasets and displaying the data

Equipment

Computerized Tomography (CT)

- Rotating detectors are positioned opposite an X-ray source. Detectors record the intensity of X-rays that have passed through the body. A three-dimensional image is generated from a series of two-dimensional X-ray images taken around a single axis of rotation. The thicker the slice, the less detail acquired. Slices are made when the x-ray tube rotates in a circle around the patient. Each slice is divided into a matrix of voxels

- Based on the X-ray attenuations obtained from many different angles, a cross-sectional image of the body can be calculated. The linear attenuation coefficient of each 2-D pixel is measured. Pixel values are quantified in Hounsfield Units (HU), also called CT numbers. The Hounsfield scale is calibrated (1000 HU for bone, 0 HU for water and -1000 HU for air)

- Adjustments can be made in the final images for black to white (gray scale of the images). This is referred to as window "width" and window "level". The width value represents the range of CT numbers that are displayed on a gray scale. Each value below that range will be displayed black, and each value above the range will be shown white. The "level" or "center" value determines the CT number around which the window is centered. The window level should be centered near the average CT number of the organ of interest. As window width increases, contrast decreases and the latitude (range of CT numbers imaged) increases

- CT is a good modality for the delineation of bony pathology, or to detect small nodules (especially in the lung)

Some contrast agents used in CT are:

- Aqueous Iodine for oral GI contrast
- Non-ionic iodine for vascular enhancement
- Dilute barium suspension for GI contrast

Magnetic Resonance Imaging (MR or MRI)

- A strong magnetic field is used to align atoms within the body. Radio frequency pulses are used to produce a signal or "echo" which is received back from the patient and fed into a computer to produce an image. The contrast on the MR image can be manipulated by changing the pulse sequence parameters. The most common sequences are the T1 weighted and T2 weighted spin-echo sequences. The cerebrospinal fluid (CSF) can help determine which pulse sequence was used. If the CSF is dark, it is a T1-weighted image. If the CSF is bright (high signal), then it is a T2-weighted imaged. FLAIR (Fluid Attenuated Inversion Recovery) images are T2-weighted with the CSF signal suppressed

- MRI can display high tissue contrast and is a good modality for imaging soft tissue lesions

- Some contrast agents used in MR are:

    - Barium for GI contrast – a negative contrast agent opposed to positive in CT
    - Gadolinium for vascular enhancement

Positron Emission Tomography (PET)

- PET is a nuclear medicine imaging procedure that measures metabolic functions in the body. It can identify abnormalities that may signal tumor growth. PET is used in conjunction with CT for tumor localization and treatment planning

Tumor Localization

Some of the most obvious steps are often overlooked when preparing a patient for treatment. Starting with the basics before each procedure will prevent time consuming efforts to reproduce the initial patient position

- Patient Alignment - The use of external landmarks (eyes, nose, sternal notch, xiphoid process, navel, legs) as well as the sagittal laser through middle of body can help to insure that the patient is straight on the table. The spine can be an effective way to straighten a patient when imaging is used. Adjustment of the patients hips or shoulders may be required

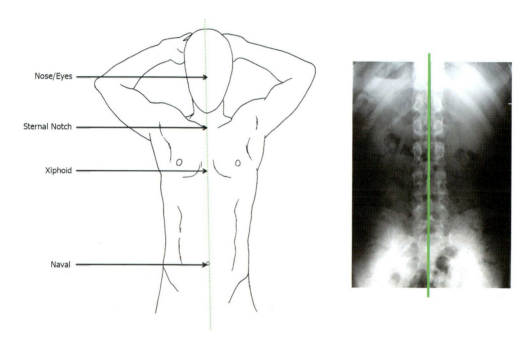

- Localization – identifying the position and extent of the tumor volume using a three dimensional coordinate system

- Coordinate System - used to describe the location of any point with respect to another known point (origin) along the x, y and z axes

- Triangulation - three landmarks whose intersection marks a single reproducible point within a patient. Three reference points can confirm patient alignment in three planes (x,y,z). Shifts can be made from this location to another location within the patient

- Isocenter - fixed point in space where the central axes of the radiation beams intersect from every angle. The gantry, table and collimators all rotate around this point. Positioning lasers are aligned to intersect at this point. Generally set at 100 cm from the radiation source for modern linear accelerators. The field size for a treatment unit is defined at the isocenter of the machine

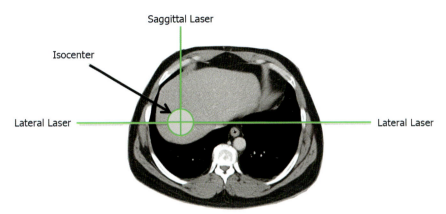

Triangulation

- Source to Skin Distance (SSD) - the distance from the radiation source to the patient's skin, usually measured using an Optical Distance Indicator (ODI) or rangefinder

    o Fixed (SSD) setup - patient is treated using a fixed distance from the radiation source (usually 100 cm) to the patient's skin surface. The patient must be moved to this same distance between each treatment

    o The advantages of SSD treatments are the ability to obtain a larger field size at a greater distance from the radiation source, and a slight increase in the percentage depth dose. The dose distribution in the patient becomes more homogeneous from entrance to exit (increased percentage of radiation within the patient relative to the percentage of the maximum entrance dose (Dmax)). However, at an increased distance it will take longer to get the same dose to a point in the patient

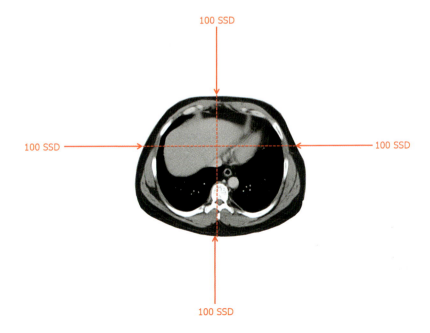

- Source to Axis Distance (SAD) - distance from the radiation source to the isocenter of the treatment machine. When the gantry rotates around the patient, the SSD continually changes; however, the SAD is at a fixed distance and will not change (usually 100 cm)
    - Isocentric (SAD) setup - the isocenter is established at some reference point inside the patient. The gantry (source) rotates around this point (axis). Since the field size is defined at the isocenter, the collimated field size is defined by the field size set inside the patient and not the field size on the skin surface as seen in the non-isocentric, SSD treatment setup. (SAD = SSD + depth to isocenter)
    - An advantage of SAD treatments is that once the isocenter for the treatment has been established, there is no movement of the patient for each of the subsequent treatment fields. Less movement between fields lowers the chance of treatment errors because of positioning variations during patient movement

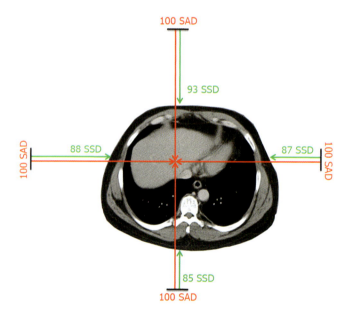

Geometric Parameters and Patient Measurement

- Magnification – field size and collimator setting are directly proportional
    - Field Size - the dimensions of a treatment field at the isocenter. A graticule (bb tray or dot tray) is a grid to assist in determining field dimensions, magnification of an image, and the central ray location. The central ray is the center of the beam where there is no divergence
    - Target = Source. The terms are interchangeable (TSD=SSD, TFD=SFD)

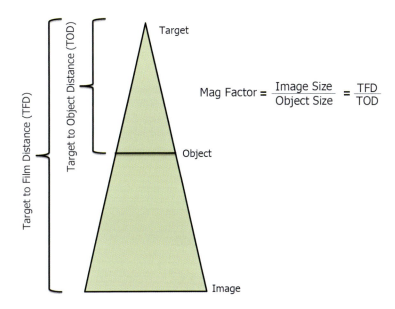

Field Magnification Examples

A patient is being treated at 115 SSD on a 100 cm SAD machine. The collimators have been set to 35 cm X 40 cm. What is the field size on the patient's skin?

$$\frac{35}{100} = \frac{x}{115} \qquad \frac{40}{100} = \frac{Y}{115}$$

$$100x = 4025 \qquad 100y = 4600$$

$$X = 40.25 \qquad Y = 46$$

(40.3 cm X 46 cm)

A field size measures 42 cm X 36 cm at 110 cm away from the radiation source. What is the field size at 100 cm?

$$\frac{42}{110} = \frac{x}{100} \qquad \frac{36}{110} = \frac{Y}{100}$$

$$110x = 4200 \qquad 110y = 3600$$

$$X = 38.18 \qquad Y = 32.72$$

$$\boxed{38.2 \text{ cm X } 32.7 \text{ cm}}$$

A patient is being treated with a 45 cm X 42 cm field size on the skin. The largest field setting is a 40 cm X 40 cm at 100 SAD. What should the SSD read on the skin to achieve this field size? (HINT: 45 cm is the larger of the two dimensions, so the only calculation needed is the larger field to get the required SSD)

$$\frac{45}{X} = \frac{40}{100}$$

$$40x = 4500$$

$$X = 112.5$$

$$\boxed{SSD = 112.5}$$

A localization film was taken at 109 cm Source to Film Distance (SFD). A 3.5 cm magnification ring was placed on the patient's skin. The same ring measured 4.2 cm on the film. What is the distance of the magnification ring from the source?

$$\frac{4.2}{109} = \frac{3.5}{X}$$

$$4.2x = 381.5$$

$$X = 90.8$$

$$\boxed{90.8 \text{ cm}}$$

A block measures 7 cm X 11 cm on a digital image taken 105 cm from the source. The block tray is 45 cm from the source. What is the actual size of the block?

$$\frac{7}{105} = \frac{X}{45} \qquad \frac{11}{105} = \frac{Y}{45}$$

$$105x = 315 \qquad 105y = 495$$

$$X = 3 \qquad Y = 4.7$$

$$\boxed{3 \text{ cm X } 4.7 \text{ cm}}$$

- o Distortion is a change in size, shape, or appearance. Shape changes when the image is not parallel with the image plane (like a shadow). Direct proportions <u>do not apply</u> when the beam is not perpendicular to the image plane

- Patient Separation (thickness) – the measurement of patient thickness from the point of beam entry to the point of beam exit. Separation can be measured directly using calipers or indirectly by using ODI (rangefinder) readings

  - o To measure patient separation indirectly, set 100 SSD to the surface of the skin and use a ruler to measure the distance from the top of the table to the lateral laser crossing at the skins surface

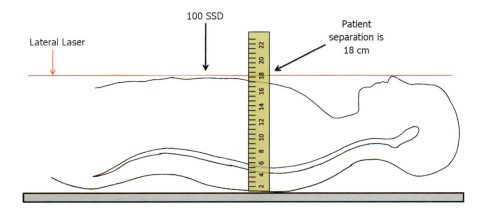

SAD, SSD, and Separation Examples

A patient's thickness is 36 cm. The SSD on the anterior surface reads 88 cm. What should the posterior SSD read if the patient is on a 100 cm SAD machine?

100 cm SAD − 88 cm SSD = 12 cm

36 cm thickness − 12 cm = 24 cm

100 cm SAD − 24 cm = 76 cm SSD

76 cm PA SSD

If the same patient is on an 80 SAD machine, what would the AP and PA SSD's read?

80 cm SAD − 12 cm depth = 68 AP SSD

36 cm thickness − 12 cm = 24 cm

80 cm SAD − 24 cm = 56 cm SSD

68 cm AP SSD
56 cm PA SSD

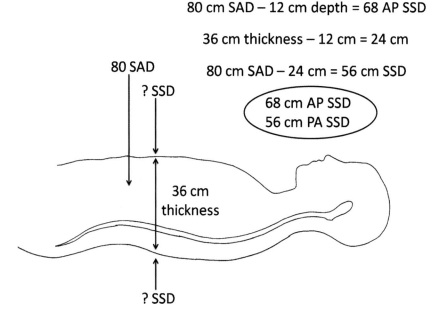

A patient is supine on the treatment table and the AP SSD reads 87 cm. If the isocenter is moved 2 cm posterior in the patient, what is the new AP SSD?

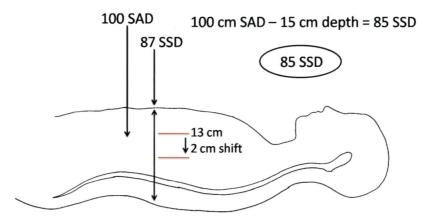

- Inverse Square – a mathematical relationship that describes the change in beam intensity caused by the divergence of the beam. This is NOT a direct proportion like field size magnification because it takes into account the increased **area** of the beam opposed to the perimeter dimensions like field size

    o As the radiation beam diverges away from the source, the area increases and the intensity decreases

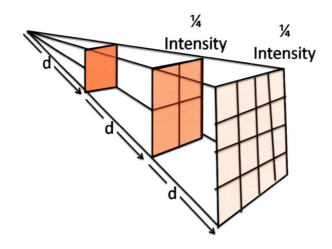

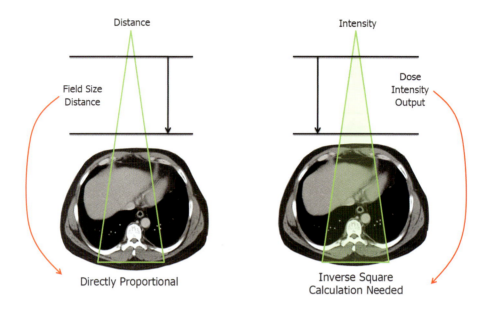

Inverse Square Examples

$$\frac{I_1}{I_2} = \left[\frac{(d_2)}{(d_1)}\right]^2$$

If the dose delivered at 100 cm is 100cGy, what is the dose at 115 cm if only the distance changes?

$$\frac{100 \text{ cGy}}{I_2} = \left[\frac{(115)}{(100)}\right]^2$$

$$\frac{100 \text{ cGy}}{I_2} = \left[1.15\right]^2$$

$$100 \text{ cGy} = 1.32 \, (I_2)$$

$$\boxed{76 \text{ cGy} = I_2}$$

The output of the machine is 200 cGy/minute at 110 cm away from the source. At what distance will the output be 400 cGy/minute?

$$\frac{200 \text{ cGy}}{400 \text{ cGy}} = \left[\frac{(d_2)}{(110)}\right]^2$$

$$0.5 = \left[\frac{(d_2)}{(110)}\right]^2$$

$$\sqrt{0.5} = \left[\frac{(d_2)}{(110)}\right]$$

$$77.8 \text{ cm} = (d_2)$$

A person receives 50 cGy/minute at 2 feet from the source. How far away does this person have to move to receive 20 cGy/minute?

$$\frac{50 \text{ cGy}}{20 \text{ cGy}} = \left[\frac{(d_2)}{(2)}\right]^2$$

$$2.5 = \left[\frac{(d_2)}{(2)}\right]^2$$

$$\sqrt{2.5} = \left[\frac{(d_2)}{(2)}\right]$$

$$3.16 \text{ ft} = (d_2)$$

A person receives 10 cGy/minute at three feet away from the source. What dose is received per second if the person moves to nine feet away from the source?

$$\frac{10 \text{ cGy}}{I_2} = \left[\frac{(9)}{(3)}\right]^2$$

$$\frac{10 \text{ cGy}}{I_2} = 9$$

$$10 \text{ cGy} = 9(I_2)$$

$$1.1 \text{ cGy/min} = I_2$$

$$\frac{1.1 \text{ cGy/min}}{60 \text{ seconds}}$$

$$\boxed{0.018 \text{ cGy/sec}}$$

- Mayneord's F (factor) - a special application of Inverse Square that is rarely used in clinical practice. Does not account for changes in scatter due to field size changes with beam divergence. It approximates the new percentage depth dose for a change in distance from the source

- Change in distance has a much greater effect on radiation output than a change in field size. The field size change with distance is slight (directly proportional) compared to beam intensity (inverse square). Mayneord's F formula can be used to estimate the change in percentage depth dose when the distance is either extended or shortened and the field size setting remains the same. The Mayneord's F equation is:

$$\text{New PDD} = \text{Old PDD} \times \frac{(\text{Old SSD} + \text{tx depth})^2 (\text{New SSD} + \text{dmax})^2}{(\text{Old SSD} + \text{dmax})^2 (\text{New SSD} + \text{tx depth})^2}$$

Mayneord's F Examples

A patient is treated with an 8 cm X 15 cm field at 80 cm SSD to a depth of 5 cm using a 6 MV linear accelerator. The percentage depth dose at 5 cm for a 10.5 equivalent square field size is 61%. If the distance is extended to 100 cm SSD, what is the new percentage depth dose?

$$\text{New PDD} = (0.61) \frac{(80+5)^2 (100+1.5)^2}{(80+1.5)^2 (100+5)^2}$$

$$\text{New PDD} = (0.61) \frac{(7225)(10302.3)}{(6642.3)(11025)}$$

$$\text{New PDD} = (0.61)(1.016)$$

$$\text{New PDD} = \boxed{0.62 = 62\%}$$

Beam Characteristics

Beam profiles, percent depth dose curves, and isodose curves are all graphic representations of the dose from a radiation source

- Beam profiles illustrate radiation intensity across the beam at a given depth

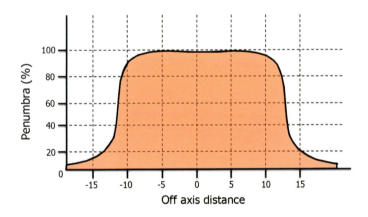

- Percent depth dose curves are typically plotted as a percentage of dose deposited at a depth. They are normalized to percent depth dose at dmax (100%)

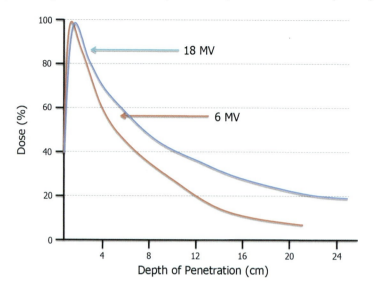

- Isodose curves show the dose that is delivered at various depths across a beam. Isodose lines connect points having the same dose

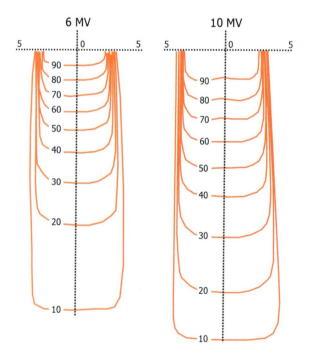

- Penumbra is the area of decreased dose at the edge of the beam. It is the dose measured between the 20% and 80% isodose lines. Lower energy beams have more penumbra due to lateral scatter
    - Physical Penumbra - a sum of the dose contributed from a portion of the primary beam at the field edge and scatter radiation. Physical penumbra is determined by geometric penumbra and lateral scatter
    - Geometric Penumbra - defines the width of the beam's penumbra and is independent of field size. It is dependent on source size, source to skin distance (SSD), and source collimator distance (SCD). Geometric penumbra <u>increases</u> with: depth, SSD, and source size. It <u>decreases</u> with an increase in SCD
        - Geometric penumbra can be calculated with the equation:

$$P = \frac{s(SAD - SCD)}{SCD} = \frac{s(SSD + d - SCD)}{SCD}$$

        - P = geometric penumbra (cm)
        - s = source size (cm)
        - SAD = Source to Axis Distance (cm)
        - SCD = Source to Collimator Distance (cm)
        - SSD = Source to Skin Distance (cm)

Geometric Penumbra Examples

A cobalt-60 source size is 1.5 cm. The patient is treated at 100 cm SSD to a depth of 6 cm. The source collimator (diaphragm) distance is 30 cm. What is the size of the penumbra on the patient's skin?

$$\text{Penumbra} = \frac{1.5\ (100\ SSD + 0\ cm\ depth\ (skin\ surface) - 30\ cm\ SCD)}{30\ cm\ SCD}$$

$$\frac{1.5\ cm\ (70)}{30\ cm\ SCD}$$

$$\boxed{3.5\ cm}$$

Dose Calculations and Factors

Machine output data

- Output - referred to as the dose rate of the machine. It is the amount of radiation exposure produced by a treatment machine using a specified reference field size (usually 10cm x 10cm) at a specified reference distance (100 cm from the source) and at a specified depth in a specified material (usually phantom). When performing dose calculations it is important to note where the machine output is measured (calibration point). Any change in distance from the source or change in field size from the calibration point must be adjusted using the correct factors

- Dose maximum (dmax) - the depth of maximum buildup where 100% of the dose is deposited. This the depth of electronic equilibrium (amount of energy lost is equal to the energy gained)

Dose Calculation Factors

- Field Size Factor (FSF) (Sc, Sp)

    - Collimator Scatter (Sc) - the ratio of the dose rate of a given field size to the dose rate of the reference field size measured in air. The collimator scatter factor allows for the change in scatter as the collimator setting changes. The collimator scatter factor is usually normalized or referenced to a 10 cm X 10 cm field size. This means that the collimator scatter factor for a 10 cm X 10 cm field size is 1.0. The collimator scatter factor will be greater than 1.0 for field sizes larger than 10 cm X 10 cm because of an increase in scatter as the collimator setting is increased. The collimator scatter factor will be less than 1.0 for field sizes smaller than 10 cm X 10 cm because of a decrease in scatter as the collimator setting is decreased

    - Phantom Scatter (Sp) - scatter from the patient. This factor is derived by measuring machine output in a phantom (tissue equivalent). If the known collimator scatter factor is removed from the dose measured with a reference field size (10 cm x 10 cm) and the new field size, the remaining change in dose is due to phantom scatter. Phantom scatter increases with increasing field size. It is dependent on the field size for patient treatment. If blocking is used, phantom scatter is dependent on the equivalent field size of the blocked field

Field Size Factor

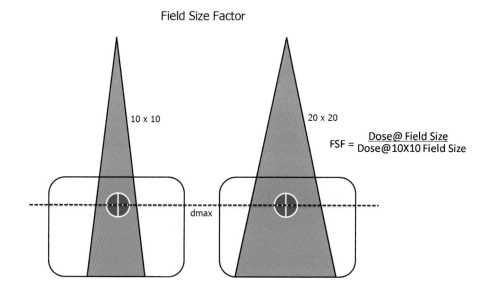

Collimator Scatter Factor Example

A 10 cm X 10 cm field size delivers 0.99 cGy/monitor unit at 100 SAD in air. If a 15 cm X 15 cm delivers 1.02 cGy/monitor unit at 100 SAD in air, what is the percentage increase of scatter from the 15 cm X 15 cm collimator setting as compared to the 10 cm X 10cm?

$$\frac{1.02}{.99} = 1.03 = \boxed{3\%}$$

- Equivalent Square (open and blocked)
    - To simplify the many combinations of field sizes, the area treated can be equated to the same area within a square field. This is called the equivalent square of the rectangular field size. Equating rectangular fields to an equivalent square reduces the number of rectangular fields that must be measured to obtain the output reading

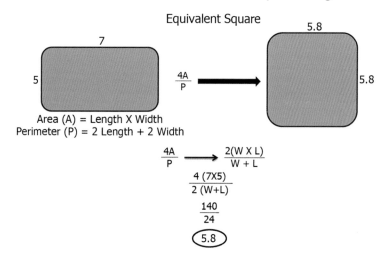

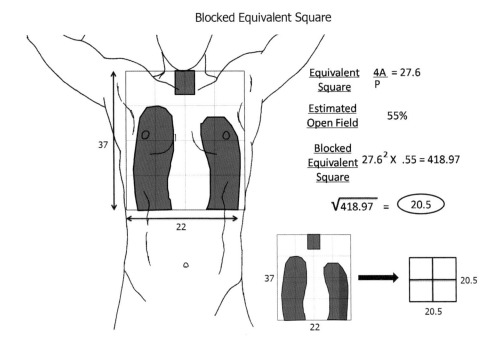

Blocked Equivalent Square

Equivalent Square: $\dfrac{4A}{P} = 27.6$

Estimated Open Field: 55%

Blocked Equivalent Square: $27.6^2 \times .55 = 418.97$

$\sqrt{418.97} = 20.5$

Equivalent Square Examples

Find the equivalent square of a 9 cm X 17 cm field.

$$\dfrac{4(9 \times 17)}{2(9+17)} = \dfrac{612}{52} = 11.76$$

11.8 cm X 11.8 cm

Find the blocked equivalent square of a 12 cm X 12 cm that has a 4 cm X 6 cm block.

$$\sqrt{(12 \times 12) - (4 \times 6)} = 10.95$$

11 cm X 11 cm

* 12 X 12 = open area
* 4 X 6 = blocked area
* 11 X 11 = blocked equivalent square

- Back Scatter Factor (BSF) and Peak Scatter Factor (PSF)

    o BSF is the ratio of the dose rate with a scattering medium to the dose rate at the same point without a medium (in air) at dmax. Adjusts the dose rate in air to dose rate in tissue (if the calibration is done in air). BSF is the Tissue Air Ratio (TAR) at dmax. For superficial and orthovoltage energies, dmax is on the skin surface. For megavoltage energies it is below the skin surface. The term Peak Scatter Factor is preferred for high energies to describe the forward, lateral and backscatter which reach equilibrium below the skin surface (dmax). As field size increases, BSF increases due to more scatter. As radiation energy increases, the measured depth of dmax may shift deeper for large field sizes due to increase in patient and collimation scatter

Back Scatter Factor

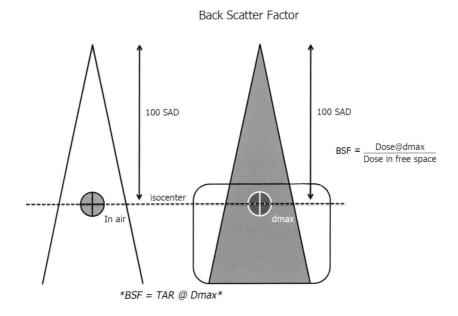

BSF = TAR @ Dmax

Back Scatter Example

The output (dose rate) for a Cobalt - 60 source in air is 1.02 cGy/minute at 100.5 cm for a 15 cm X 15 cm field. The back scatter factor for a 15 cm X 15 cm field size at dmax (100.5 cm) is 1.1. What is the dose rate in tissue at dmax?

$$1.02 \text{ cGy/min} \times 1.1 = \boxed{1.12 \text{ cGy/min}}$$

- Scatter Air Ratio (SAR)
    - SAR is the ratio of the scattered dose at a given point to the dose in free space at the same point. SAR is used to determine the contribution of scatter to a point of calculation in a field. SAR is especially useful for irregular fields as the contribution of scatter radiation to the primary radiation beam will not be equal from all sides
- Percentage Depth Dose (PDD) (%DD)
    - PDD is used with SSD technique. The ratio of the absorbed dose at a given depth to the absorbed dose at a fixed reference point (usually dmax)
    - PDD is dependent on the following factors:
        - PDD increases with an increase in beam energy (quality)
        - PDD decreases with an increase in depth past dmax
        - PDD increases with an increase in field size
        - PDD increases with an increase in SSD

Percentage Depth Dose

$$PDD = \frac{Dose@depth}{Dose@dmax}$$

Dmax = 100% of Dose

Percentage Depth Dose Example

A patient is receiving 300 cGy to a spinal cord lesion at the 78.5% DD line. What is the dose delivered at dmax?

$$\frac{300 \text{ cGy}}{0.785} = 382 \text{ cGy}$$

The dose at dmax is 112 cGy with a 15 cm X 15 cm field size and a SSD of 100. If the percentage depth dose is 67% at 10 cm with a 15 cm X 15 cm field size at 100 cm SSD, what dose is delivered at 10 cm?

Dose at dmax = tumor dose /PDD. Therefore dose at dmax * PDD = tumor dose

$$112 \text{ cGy} \times 0.67 = \boxed{75 \text{ cGy}}$$

The dose rate at 100.5 cm in air (dmax) is 1.04 cGy/monitor unit for a 15 cm x 15 cm field. The backscatter factor for a 15 cm X 15 cm is 1.01 and the % dd is 0.67 at a depth of 11 cm. How many monitor units are needed to deliver 300 cGy to a 15 cm X 15 cm field at 11 cm?

$$\text{Tx time or MU} = \frac{\text{Tumor dose}}{(\text{dose rate in air @ 100.5 cm for collimator setting})(\text{BSF})(\text{PDD})}$$

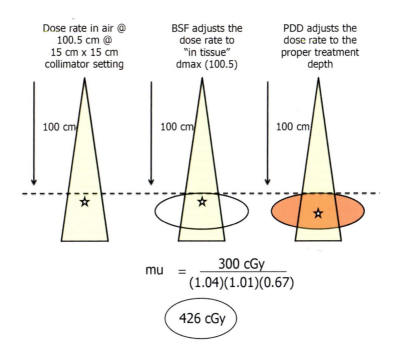

$$mu = \frac{300 \text{ cGy}}{(1.04)(1.01)(0.67)}$$

$$\boxed{426 \text{ cGy}}$$

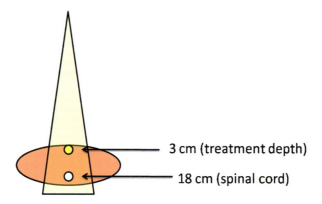

200 cGy is prescribed through a single field to the treatment depth of 3 cm. The PDD at 3 cm is .95. The physician wants to know the dose received at the spinal cord at a depth of 18 cm in the patient. The PDD for this field at a depth of 18 cm is .44.

$$\frac{200 \text{ cGy}}{.95} \times .44 = \boxed{92.6 \text{cGy}}$$

- Note that the dose is measured at two different depths (two distances from the source) and the distance from the source to skin surface remains constant. This means calculating dose to another point on the central axis (CAX) with the same field size becomes a simple ratio of the percentage depth dose

- Tissue Air Ratio (TAR)
  - TAR is used for SAD setups. It is the ratio of the absorbed dose at a given depth in a phantom to the absorbed dose at the same point in free space. TAR adjusts the dose rate from air to tissue and treatment depth
  - TAR is dependent upon the following factors:
    - TAR increases with an increase in beam energy (quality)
    - TAR decreases with an increase in depth past dmax
    - TAR increases with an increase in field size
    - TAR is NOT dependent upon SSD

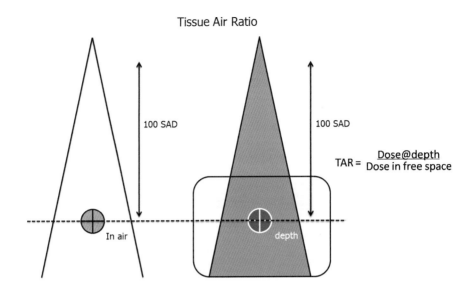

- Tissue Maximum Ratio (TMR)
  - TMR is the ratio of the absorbed dose at a given depth in a phantom to the absorbed dose at the same point at a reference point of dmax
  - TMR is similar to TAR, but in tissue at a specified point. TMR was developed because of the difficulty of measuring high energy output in air
    - TMR is related to TAR by using the formula:

$$TAR = TMR \times BSF$$

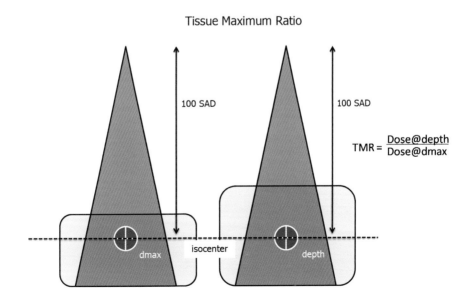

- Tissue Phantom Ratio (TPR)
    - TPR is the ratio of the absorbed dose at a given depth in phantom to the absorbed dose at the same point at a given reference depth (e.g. 5 cm, 10 cm)
    - The reference depth will not change with field size like TMR (depth of dmax can be influenced by field size for higher energies)
        - TMR is TPR at the reference depth of dmax

Tissue Phantom Ratio

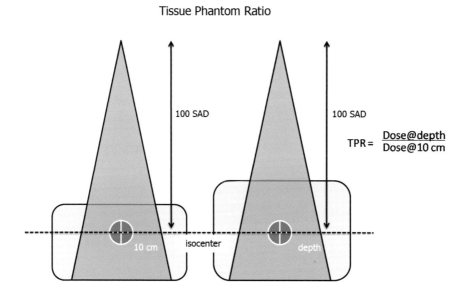

TAR, TMR, and TPR Examples

The dose rate at 100 cm in air is 1 cGy/monitor unit for the calibration field. The collimator scatter factor for an 8 cm X 8 cm is 0.99 and the TAR is 0.96 at a depth of 3 cm. How many monitor units are needed to deliver 300 cGy to an 8 cm X 8 cm field at 3 cm?

$$mu = \frac{\text{tumor dose}}{(\text{dose rate in air @ 100 cm (10 X 10)})(Sc)(TAR)}$$

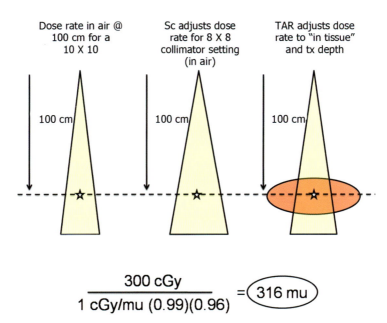

$$\frac{300 \text{ cGy}}{1 \text{ cGy/mu }(0.99)(0.96)} = 316 \text{ mu}$$

A patient is treated isocentrically (100 cm SAD) with parallel opposed ports, both at a depth of 10 cm, 15 x15 cm field size. The dose rate at 100 cm is 0.01 Gy/mu at dmax in tissue for the calibration field size. The field size factor is 1.023 for a 15 x15 field and the TMR is 0.75 for this setup. Find the number of monitor units required for one field if the two fields are equally weighted and the total tumor dose is 1.8 Gy daily.

$$mu = \frac{\text{tumor dose}}{(\text{dose rate in tissue @ 100 cm (10 X 10)})(FSF)(TMR)}$$

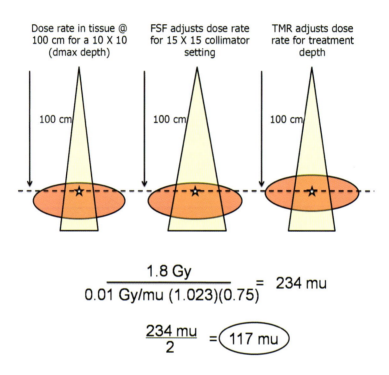

$$\frac{1.8 \text{ Gy}}{0.01 \text{ Gy/mu } (1.023)(0.75)} = 234 \text{ mu}$$

$$\frac{234 \text{ mu}}{2} = \boxed{117 \text{ mu}}$$

TMR and TPR problems are essentially the same. The TMR is a TPR measured at dmax

- TAR, TMR and TPR are all measured at a specified distance from the source, usually 100 cm. The depth of overlying tissue may change, but the distance to the point of calculation (isocenter) remains constant. For this reason when you want to compute the dose to another point on the central axis, you must apply a field size correction (field size is defined at 100 cm) and an inverse square correction because the new point will not be located at isocenter

A 13 cm X 13 cm equivalent square field is used to deliver a dose of 100 cGy to a point at 12 cm depth, 100 SAD. What is the dose delivered to a point at 10 cm depth on the central axis (CAX)?

$$\text{Convert field size -} \quad \frac{13 \text{ cm}}{100 \text{ cm}} = \frac{X}{98 \text{ cm}} \longrightarrow X \approx 12.5$$

$$\text{New dose @ 10 cm} = \frac{(100 \text{ cGy})(98^2)}{(0.59)(100^2)} \quad 0.65$$

$$\text{Dose @10 cm} = \boxed{105.8 \text{ cGy}}$$

- 100 cGy = original dose for 13 x 13 @ 10 cm depth
- 0.59 = TMR for 13 x 13
- 98 = source to new point distance
- 100 = source to old point distance
- 0.65 = TMR for 12.5 x 12.5

Dose Calculations and Factors

- Off Axis Factor (OAF) - the highest dose is at the CAX of the beam, and the dose decreases with greater distance from the CAX. For this reason a flattening filter is used in the treatment machine to create a uniform dose across the field. Measurements must be made to determine the ratio of the dose at the central axis to the dose off of the central axis. This ratio is called an off-axis ratio or factor and must be incorporated when calculating the dose to a point off the central axis
    - The central ray of the beam has NO divergence. It can be "hotter" than the rest of the field, but a flattening filter helps to even out the dose over the entire field. The flattening filter evens out the dose by attenuating the radiation beam. The thickest part of the flattening filter is lined up with the strongest photon beam to help to deliver an evenly distributed dose

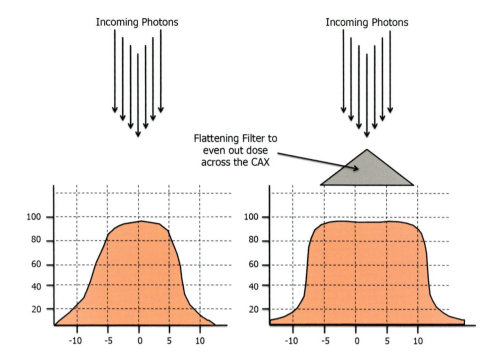

- Reasons an Off Axis Factor may be used for dose calculation:
    - A half beam block on the central axis
    - A block is placed over the central axis

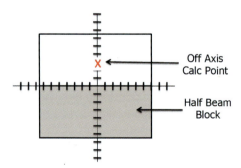

- Physical Wedges and Compensators
    - A wedge or compensator filter alters the isodose patterns. The compensator filter is individually produced for each patient and alters the patterns so that they are tailored to the patient anatomy. The wedge is defined by the tilt in the isodose lines

- The wedge angle is defined as the angle between a line drawn perpendicular to the central axis and the specified isodose curve or depth

- The addition of a wedge will always increase the number of monitor units required to deliver a dose to a specific point using a specific field size

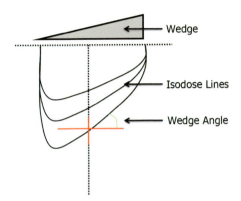

- The hinge angle formula is used to predict the appropriate wedge based on the angle between the central axis of two beams (hinge angle). Based on the concept that the thicker end of the wedges (heels) should be oriented toward one another to correct for the overlap region. The hinge angle formula is not always accurate due to other factors such as tissue inhomogeneities and surface irregularities

Wedge angle (Θ) = 90-(Hinge angle /2)

Wedge Angle Examples

If the hinge angle between two beams is 90 degrees, what is the wedge angle that should be used?

$$90 - (90/2) = \boxed{45° \text{ wedge}}$$

The wedge factor for a 45 degree wedge for the field size and depth of interest is 0.56. The original open field required 162 monitor units to deliver 100 cGy. What are the new monitor units needed when the wedge is placed in the path of the beam?

$$\frac{162 \text{ mu}}{0.56} = \boxed{289 \text{ mu}}$$

- Dynamic Wedges
    - The collimator jaw position and movement can cause a wedge effect
    - There are no attenuation factors (dependent on the position of the moving jaw and the number of delivered monitor units)
    - Dynamic wedges require a continuous QA program to monitor output
- Transmission Filters
    - Transmission filters allow a specified percentage of the beam to pass through the blocked area
    - Transmission filter example: a 50% transmission filter would allow 50% of the prescribed dose to exit through the transmission block so that the area below would receive half of the prescribed dose throughout the treatment. Useful in the treatment of radiosensitive organs such as the liver where surrounding tissues can tolerate more than the area below the block
- Tray Factor
    - The tray transmission factor (tray factor) defines how much of the radiation is transmitted through a block tray. When the beam of radiation hits the tray, some of the radiation will be attenuated by the tray. The radiation not attenuated by the tray will pass through and continue to the patient. To correctly calculate a monitor unit or time setting, the amount of radiation transmitted through the tray must be measured. The physicist takes two measurements: the first measurement is with the tray in the path of the beam, while the second measurement is without the tray in the path of the beam. The ratio of these two measurements is known as the tray transmission factor. A tray factor will always cause the output to decrease. Therefore, the monitor units (mu) will increase when compared to the mu's for an open field to deliver the prescribed dose

Tray Factor Example

An open field is measured and a plexiglass block tray is added into the path of the beam. The attenuation tray factor is 1.031. If the ouput measured without the tray is 200 cGy/minute, what is the output at the same distance and field dimensions with the tray added?

$$\frac{200 \text{ cGy/min}}{1.031} = \boxed{194 \text{ cGy/min}}$$

- Bolus
    - Bolus is a tissue equivalent material that can be used to fill a body cavity, or be placed on the skin to increase surface dose (bring dmax closer to the skin surface)
- Inhomogeneity Correction Factors and Equivalent Depth
    - A simplified method to calculate dose through different mediums is to assign a correction factor for tissue types based on their electron density. Electron density for bone depends on how compact the bone is; spongy bone may have an electron density only 1.1 times the density of water and very compact bone's density is up to 1.65 times the density of water. If the beam passes through tissue less dense than water, such as lung or an air cavity, the thickness of this tissue is multiplied by a number less than 1.0; the resulting equivalent depth is less than the actual depth. Adding the tissue thickness and multiplying by the appropriate correction factors results in the equivalent depth in tissue. This method does not take into account the effects seen at the interface between tissues of differing densities. This effect is especially important when dealing with high LET radiations. Sophisticated algorithms have been developed for treatment planning systems to more accurately predict dose as it travels through tissue inhomogenieties
        - Typical Correction Factors:
            - Soft tissue – 1.0
            - Bone – 1.3
            - Air – 0.33
    - To get an equivalent depth, measure the length of each medium, multiply by the correction factors, and add together. This number will give you the equivalent depth of the treated area

Equivalent Depth Example

What is the equivalent depth for a tumor when the radiation beam passes through: 3 cm of soft tissue, 1 cm of bone, and 4 cm of air?

$$3 \text{ cm}(1.0) + 1 \text{ cm}(1.3) + 4 \text{ cm}(0.33) = \boxed{5.62 \text{ cm}}$$

Treatment Delivery

- Information required before first treatment

    o Pathology report, informed consent with appropriate signatures, radiation prescription with physician signature, and a complete and approved treatment plan

- Contents of a prescription

    o Anatomic site, total tumor dose, dose per fraction, number of fractions, fractionation schedule (once a day, B.I.D., Q.O.D), protraction (time over which the total dose is delivered), beam energy, and treatment plan

- Contents of a treatment plan

    o Treatment volume – generally larger than the target volume, encompasses the additional margins around the target volume to allow for limitations of the treatment technique

    o The International Commission of Radiation Units and Measurements (ICRU) 50 definitions:

    - Gross Tumor Volume (GTV): Palpable or visible extent of tumor

    - Clinical Target Volume (CTV): GTV plus local margins for subclinical disease or regions of presumed microscopic disease

    - Planning Target Volume (PTV): CTV plus margins for treatment reproducibility factors such as patient and organ movement, respiration, and daily setup. Excludes margin for beam penumbra

    - Treated Volume: Volume enclosed by an isodose surface (e.g. 95% isodose), selected and specified by radiation oncologist as being appropriate to achieve the purpose of treatment

    - Irradiated Volume: Tissue volume which receives a dose that is considered significant in relation to normal tissue tolerance

    - Organs at Risk: Normal tissues whose radiation sensitivity may significantly influence treatment planning and/or prescribed dose

Treatment Volumes

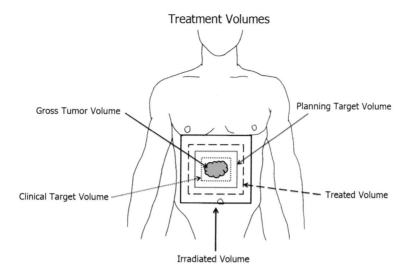

- Number of fields – the number of fields is determined by the tolerance doses of critical structures located near the tumor. Each field will deliver a portion of the prescribed dose allowing the tumor to receive the full dose while the critical structures and the healthy tissue around the tumor receive as little dose as possible

- Fixed versus rotational fields - the difference is whether or not the gantry is moving while the beam is on. Fixed means the angle is set, the beam is on, then the beam turns off and the gantry moves to the next angle. Rotational is where the gantry starts at certain angle and depending on the prescription dose and the dose rate, the gantry will stop and the beam will turn off at a certain angle

- Field weighting - dose is distributed unequally (weighted) from each of the fields. Useful when a tumor is not midline, or to limit the dose through a beam

- Beam modifiers – includes blocks, compensators, and bolus

- Field orientation – dependent on tumor location and critical structures to be missed

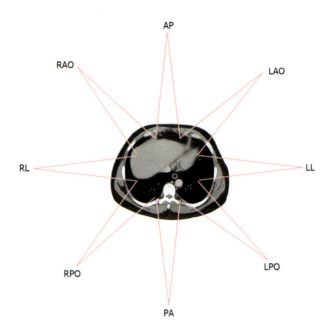

- o Energy and machine used
    - Dmax is known as the depth of maximum equilibrium, it is the depth at which electronic equilibrium occurs for photon beam, and it depends on the energy of the beam

Beam Energy	≈ Dmax Depth (cm)
200 KeV	0.0
1.25 MV	0.5
4 MV	1.0
6 MV	1.5
10 MV	2.5
18 MV	3.5
24 MV	4.0

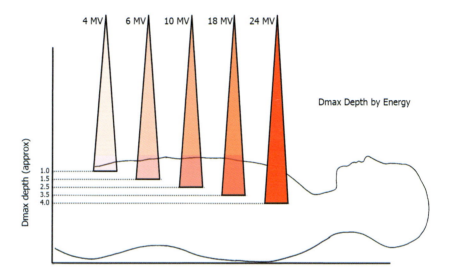

Dmax Depth by Energy

- The prescription must be rewritten and treatment plan reviewed if:
    - Field size is reduced or changed, fractionation changes, total dose changes, beam energy or orientation changes

Treatment Chart and Electronic Medical Record (EMR)

- Patient's radiation history and a legal record of their treatments

Date	Elapsed Days	Tx #	Therapist	AP mu's	PA mu's	Daily Dose	Total Dose
8/15	0	1	MS AV	210	176	180	180
8/16	1	2	avja	210	176	180	360
8/19	4	3	avja	210	176	180	540
8/20	5	4	avms	210	176	180	720
8/21	6	5	MS AV	210	176	180	900
8/22	7	6	av	210	176	180	1080
8/23	8	7	JA MS	210	176	180	1260
8/26	11	8	JA MS	210	176	180	1440

- The treatment chart includes:
    - Elapsed days - On the first day of treatment there is no elapsed day (0). Every day from the start of treatment is counted. If the first treatment is on Friday and second treatment is on Monday there are 3 elapsed days (0-Friday, 1-Saturday, 2-Sunday and 3-Monday). Every day between treatments (including scheduled breaks) must be counted. Elapsed days are continued while the patient is on break and when they resume treatment to a specified area

- Treatment Number – correlates with the number of treatments that the patient receives. (1, 2, 3...). If the patient is treated twice a day, there is no new elapsed day recorded but the treatment number increases

- Monitor Unit (MU) Setting - A calculated value that identifies how long the machine must stay on to deliver a specific dose under specified conditions. Beam energy, field size, depth, and beam attenuation devices such as wedges and blocks will effect this value

- Daily Session Dose - the total radiation dose delivered to a calculation point in one session. If multiple fractions are delivered daily, time and date must be recorded

- Cumulative Dose - the sum total dose to a specified point

- Machine Parameters - energy used, gantry angles, table angle, collimator angle, field blocking, wedges, must be accurately recorded for treatment reproducibility

- Bolus - must be prescribed by the physician and include the thickness and duration (q.d. (daily) or q.o.d. (every other day)). Prescription must be changed if bolus is discontinued (D/C)

- Therapists Initials and Date – it is important to identify the individual responsible for delivering the treatment on a given day

- Surface landmarks/Photographs – can be used to assist in localization

Field Verification Techniques

- Electronic Portal Imaging Devices (EPIDS) – a flat panel x-ray detector converts x-ray images to digital images. This can be used with an x-ray tube mounted on the accelerator (kV x-ray source) or the linear accelerator head (MV x-ray source). The digital images can be saved for static review (off-line) or reviewed in real time (on-line review)

- Image Guided Radiation Therapy (IGRT) - An x-ray tube (designed for cone beam CT or kV imaging) and a flat-panel image detector are mounted on the linear accelerator. Low dose cone beam x-rays create 3D CT images (CBCT), or 2D kV x-ray images while the patient is in the treatment position. These images are matched to the original CT plan (on-line review). Coordinates are then calculated and any necessary shifts are made to align the tumor with the radiation beam. The target position is confirmed on a daily basis prior to treatment. Markers (fiducials) can be implanted or placed on or near the target to aid in localizing the target and matching the anatomy with fixed reference points

    - A Post-treatment evaluation of images (off-line review) can be performed to monitor any shifts/changes in treatment position. Movements should be minimal if the patient is positioned properly and the setup is reproducible

- Ultrasound - image visualization and registration of subcutaneous body structures or internal organs such as the prostate

Treatment Terms and Techniques

- Static - no dynamic motion during treatment (can range from a single field to multiple fields)

- Parallel Opposed Fields (POP) – two treatment fields positioned 180° apart

- Orthogonal – two treatment fields positioned 90° apart

- Multileaf Collimation (MLC)

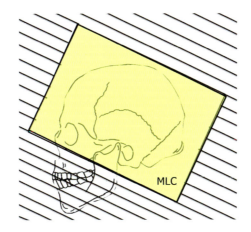

- Respiratory Gating - tracking or controlling respiratory motion during treatment. CT scans identify target volume on inspiration and exhalation

- Intensity Modulated Radiation Therapy (IMRT) - Gantry and/or collimator leaf motion and dose rate are under computer control

    o Segmental MLC (SMLC) – step and shoot. The beam turns off while the MLC leaves moves between shapes, the accelerator moves, MLC adjusts, and the beam is turned back on. These steps are repeated

"Step and Shoot"

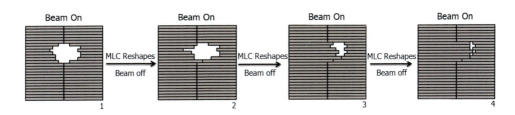

- Dynamic MLC (DMLC) – sliding window. Moves MLC leaves through one continuous beam

"Sliding Window"

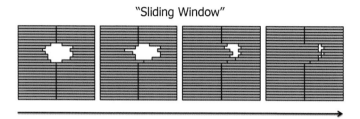

- Stereotactic Radiosurgery (SRS) – usually a single high fraction of radiation delivered to the brain

- Stereotactic Radiation Therapy (SRT) – multiple fractions of high energy radiation therapy delivered to the brain

- Stereotactic Body Radiation Therapy (SBRT) – single or small number of fractions of radiation delivered to the body (extracranial)

Services and Standards for Radiation Oncology in the United States

- National Cancer Institute (NCI) - government agency for cancer research and training under the National Institutes of Health (NIH)

- Surveillance, Epidemiology, and End Results (SEER) Program of the NCI collects and publishes cancer incidence and survival data from population-based cancer registries in the United States. It is updated annually and is provided as a public service

- Food and Drug Administration (FDA) approves all medical devices, including linear accelerators before they are marketed and sold in the United States

- American National Standards Institute (ANSI) accredits standards that are developed by organizations, government agencies, consumer groups, companies, and others. These standards ensure that products are consistent, that people use the same definitions and terms, and that products are tested the same way. Checks are performed to assure that American standards are in compliance with international standards

- Health Level 7 (HL7)- an ANSI accredited organization developing standards for exchanging clinical and administrative data

    o Examples are: demographics, financial info, scheduling, lab results, transcriptions, and medications

- Clinical Context Object Workgroup (CCOW) is an HL7 standard for multiple login through a single point

- Digital Imaging and Communications in Medicine (DICOM) – standards produced by a joint committee of the National Electrical Manufacturers Association (NEMA) and the American College of Radiology (ACR) affiliated with several international agencies
    - Publishes standards for "picture archival and communications systems" (PACS) for image storage and retrieval and assures the compatibility of computers to transfer this information

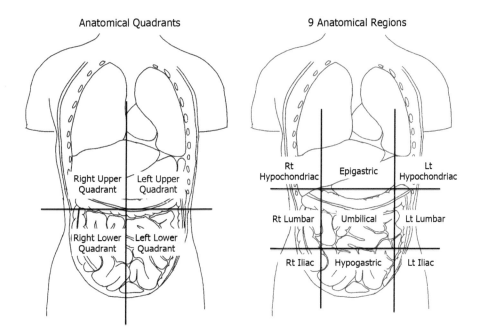

Site Specific Treatment Concepts

Head and Neck Tumors

Tumors that are located laterally and invade minimally, such as tumors of the parotid gland, can be treated using several techniques:

- Two angled beams (usually wedged to reduce the hot spots where the beams overlap) can adequately cover the tumor volume. The head can be extended back to move the level of the eyes up and out of the plane of the angled treatment fields

- An IMRT technique with constraints to avoid critical structures such as the spinal cord, opposite parotid, eyes and brain

- A lateral mixed beam using photons to reach the deeper extent of the tumor and electrons to cover the most superficial tumor volume allows the head position to remain neutral with good tumor coverage and minimal exit dose to the opposite parotid

Small, centrally located tumors, such as the pituitary gland, can be treated with multiple fields using static fields, moving arc fields, or an IMRT technique. The chin can be tucked to move the level of the eyes down and out of the treatment fields. A vertex field can be employed to reduce the dose to the temporal lobes

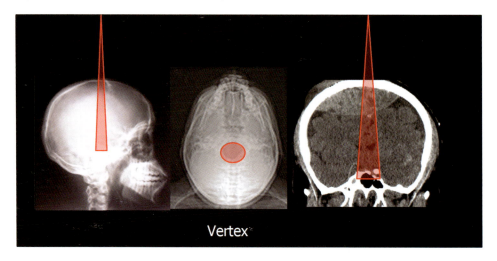

Tumors that abut the oral cavity, such as maxillary sinus tumors, may require a bite block (tongue depressor) to keep the oral tongue down and out of the treatment field. Another advantage of the bite block is to open the commissure of the lips to prevent a bolus effect in the lip folds. If the tongue is involved with tumor, the tongue depressor may be used to keep the tongue down and within the treatment field, while lifting the hard palate up and away from the tongue. The patient must be simulated and the immobilization mask made with the bite block properly positioned. The bite block should lay on the tongue and should not push the tongue into the back of the mouth

Tumors in the Chest

When positioning a patient for treatment of a tumor volume in the chest (e.g. lung, esophageal cancer), the patient may be positioned with their arms up using an immobilization device (e.g. wingboard, vaclok), or down by their sides

- Arms should be up if lateral or oblique fields are to be used for the initial fields or for boost fields, the patient should be scanned from the beginning with arms up

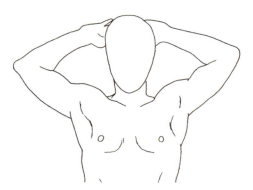

- If the entire treatment is to be delivered using an AP/PA technique, the patient can be scanned with their arms down by their sides

- The CT scan of the patient should be long enough to contour the entire lung and surrounding critical structures

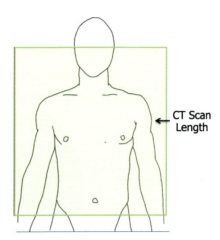

- During respiration, a tumor can move in the chest. A margin can be added to treatment fields to ensure treatment of the entire tumor volume, or the tumor can be scanned using a gated technique if this option is available

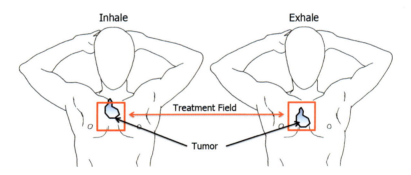

- When a tumor is not midline and is treated parallel opposed (POP), the field size or blocking may be different. The field closest to the tumor will need a larger treatment area than the field further away because of beam divergence

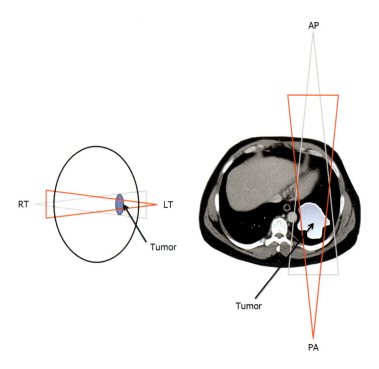

- A landmark that can be used when aligning treatment fields with DRR's is the carina. The carina is the section of the trachea that branches off into the right and left bronchus. The carina is located at T5-T6

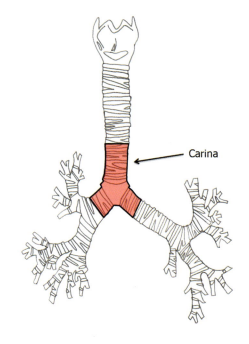

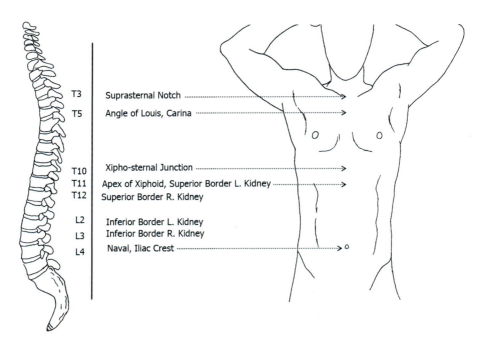

- Critical structures that should be avoided when treating esophageal and lung cancers are the spinal cord, heart, uninvolved lung, and esophagus

Tumors of the Breast

- When setting up the breast, patients must have the arm of the affected side up, but both arms may be up. A slant board can be used to compensate for the slope of the chest/lungs and also to allow the breast to fall down, and not into the neck area. An immobilization device should stabilize the arm(s) and should be indexed with the slant board

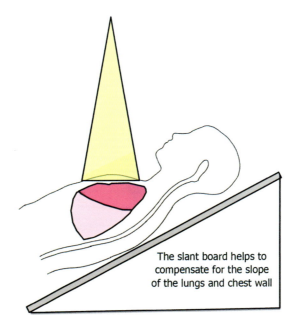

The slant board helps to compensate for the slope of the lungs and chest wall

- When setting up a breast for a CT, wires may be used to mark the breast borders and any other areas of interest. The wires can be contoured in the treatment plan to aid in field placement

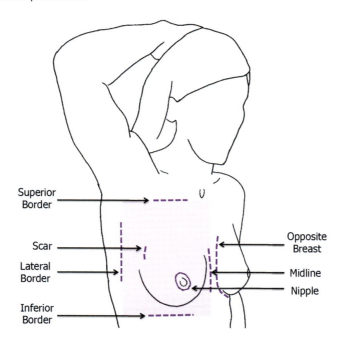

- There are multiple ways to set the tangential fields for treatment of the breast. Two commonly used techniques are the isocentric technique with non-divergent posterior borders (tangent beams are over-rotated so that the two posterior borders form a straight line along the lung interface) and the half beam technique. In the picture below, the white arrows are the central rays of the two fields. The red dots signify tattoos or marks placed on the patient to assist with daily reproducibility. The dotted red lines are the overhead and lateral lasers which coincide with the isocenter. When using the half beam technique, the central ray forms the non-divergent posterior border

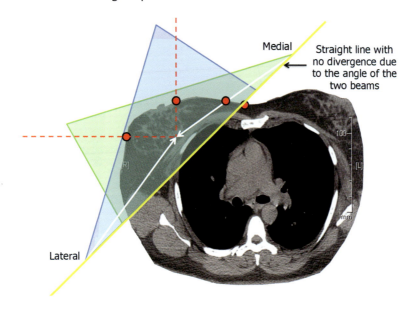

- A three field technique may be used when treating a breast if there is lymph node involvement. The three field technique adds a supraclavicular port to the original tangent fields (medial and lateral). The supraclavicular field is generally half beamed and abutted to the superior edge of the tangents. The tangents can be matched to the supraclavicular field using several methods. The top border of the tangent can be half beam blocked if an adequate field size can be achieved for the breast field using one half of the beam. Another method is to rotate the treatment couch to match the top border of the tangent to the inferior border of the supraclavicular field as illustrated below

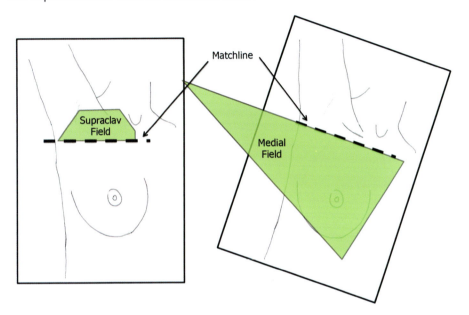

- When marking the supraclavicular field, placing more than one mark (tattoo) along the matchline will assist with daily reproducibility. It is impossible to draw a reproducible line with one dot (tattoo). With at least two dots a straight line can be drawn and the correct position can be obtained. The supraclavicular field is angled approximately 10-15 degrees away from the patient's midline to avoid the spinal cord and esophagus

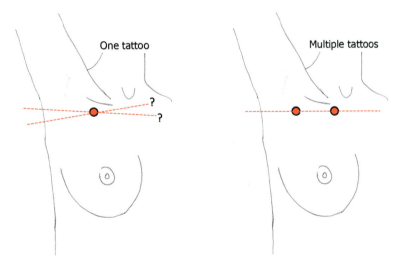

- Internal Mammary (IM) nodes are occasionally treated when there is risk of involvement. It is important that the patient is not rotated and can be positioned in a reproducible manner to avoid overlap of critical structures. The field is generally treated with electron and/or photon beams that are matched to the supraclavicular and medial border of the tangent field

Tumors of the Abdomen

- The GI tract begins at the mouth and ends at the anus. Common cancers of the GI tract are stomach, pancreatic, colorectal, and anal

- Because of the close proximity of organs in the abdomen and pelvis, some organs must be sacrificed to obtain the optimal dose to the organ of interest. IMRT can be used to reduce the amount of radiation to critical structures

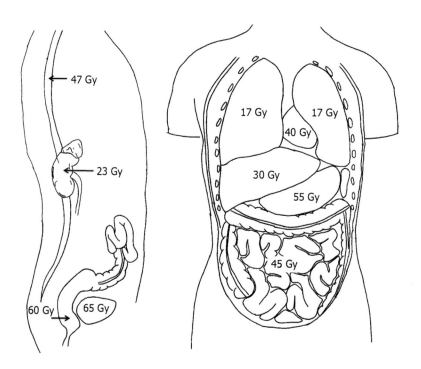

- For gastric (stomach) and pancreatic cancers, patients should be set up supine with arms above the head so oblique or lateral treatment fields can be used

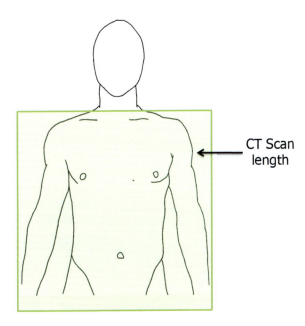

- When scanning a patient with a cancer in the abdomen, the scan should be from approximately the shoulders to the bottom of the pelvis

Tumors of the Pelvis

- When treating tumor volumes that include pelvic lymph nodes, it may be advantageous to position the patient prone on a belly board. The belly board displaces the small bowel anteriorly. For tumors that are posterior, such as rectal tumors, the prone position allows you to get a better margin around the tumor volume

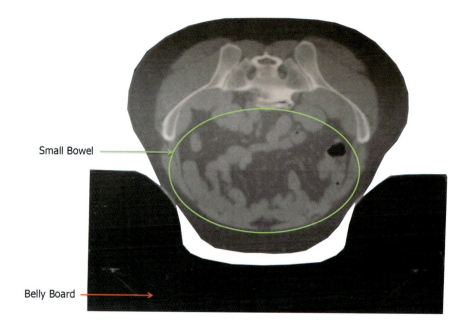

- The belly board should be indexed and the patient should be positioned in the same place on the board every day. This helps to create the same setup day after day. The belly of the patient should fall directly into the hole in the belly board, and the patient's arms should be above their head around the head cushion. The head should be positioned the same way everyday

- The prone position is not recommended for anterior tumor volumes, or patients who have difficulty lying in this position (e.g., colostomy, patient size, difficulty breathing). A patient must also lay supine if they have periaortic nodal involvement. They should be scanned with their arms up because lateral fields may be used later to avoid the kidneys. When periaortic nodes are involved, the CT scan borders should be from the carina to the bottom of the ischial tuberosity. A "frying pan" field may be used when the periaortic nodes are involved

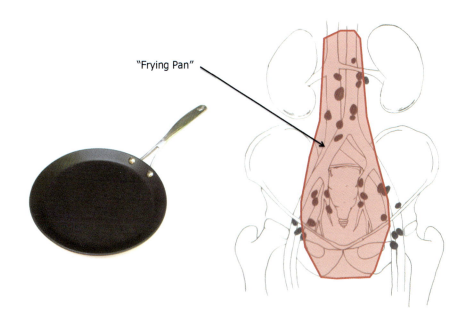

"Frying Pan"

- Markers

    o   For patients with low rectal/anal involvement a marker can be placed on the anus prior to scanning. This will help to identify the anal margin for treatment planning

    o   A vaginal marker can be placed in the vagina to identify the lowest extent of the cervix. It will stop at the external cervical os

    o   Rectal markers can also be used to identify the rectal wall for pelvic tumors (e.g. prostate or uterus)

- If inguinal nodes are to be treated the patient is usually treated supine. The legs can be immobilized in the "frog-leg" position to eliminate folds in the patients' skin that will ultimately cause skin breakdown and discomfort. Bolus can be used to bring the dose more superficially to treat the inguinal nodes

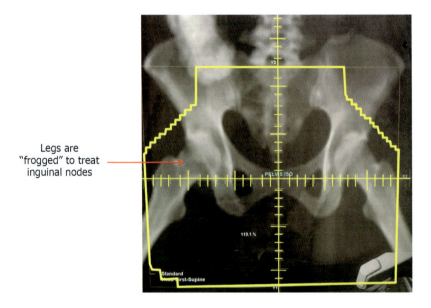

Legs are "frogged" to treat inguinal nodes

Prostate

- Immobilization and localization are extremely important when treating the prostate. A patient is to be set up supine, and a leg immobilization technique should be used (vaclok, knee cushion)

- A full bladder and an empty rectum can assist in maintaining consistency when scanning and treating a prostate patient because the prostate can be moved around in the pelvis by the bladder and rectum

    o A full bladder pushes the prostate in the same place every day and gets more of the bladder out of the treatment field

    o When the rectum is empty, it stays out of the treatment area and keeps the prostate where it should be in the pelvis

- The prostate can be treated many different ways such as: 4 field box, multiple field, and IMRT

Seminoma

- When treating a seminoma, the CT scan should be from the carina to mid-thigh. The periaortic nodes are treated with a type of frying pan technique referred to as a hockey stick

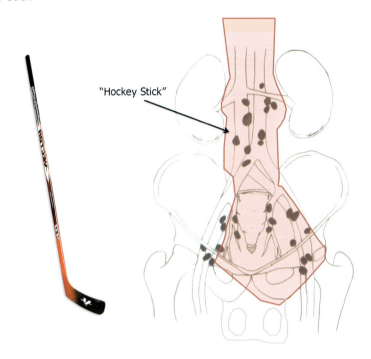

Bladder

- When scanning a bladder for treatment purposes, it should be full. When the bladder is being treated, it should be empty. This helps to ensure that the entire bladder is in the treatment field with good a margin

Tumors of the Skin

- Skin cancer is the most common form of cancer. Many skin cancer cases go unrecorded because of simple excisions

- Skin cancer is frequently treated with electrons because of the superficial qualities of electron penetration. The gantry should be parallel to the patient's skin (en face). The central ray of the beam will be perpendicular to the skin. To achieve the en face position, the gantry, collimator, and/or treatment table may be moved

- Treatment fields for skin cancer are normally set up in the treatment room (clinical setup). Lead can be used on a patient's skin to shield the surrounding skin that is not to be treated. There should be an adequate margin around the affected area. If lead is not used on the skin, cerrobend blocks can be used with the accessory mount to shape the beam to the desired shape

    o The thickness of lead (Pb) needed is determined by the energy of the electron used. Electron energy/2=mm Pb needed

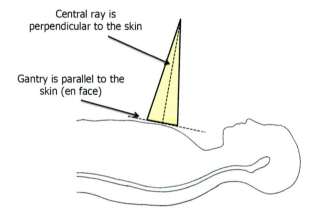

- Eye shielding - A shield can be used to block the lens of the eye from radiation. When electrons are used, opposed to low energy x-rays, a coating must be present on the shield to absorb any backscatter radiation from the electron interaction with the metal shielding. For this same reason, lead shielding (around the nose, mouth, etc) will be covered with wax, or other low Z material

- Melanoma, another type of skin cancer invades deeper into tissue and would require photon treatment

Sarcomas

- At least a 5 cm margin should be added to both the proximal and distal ends of the treatment port of a sarcoma when possible. It is important to make sure the exit dose of the beam does not exit through the opposite appendage or another body part

- The entire circumference of any appendage should never be included in the treatment field. A strip of skin is required for adequate drainage of the lymphatic system and to avoid edema

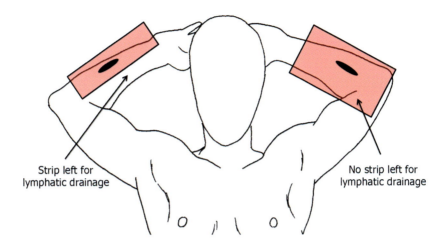

Strip left for lymphatic drainage

No strip left for lymphatic drainage

Central Nervous System

- The CNS consists of the brain and spinal cord. The treatment position is usually prone and a prone aquaplast mask is made to stabilize the head. A built up surface may be needed under the patient's torso to level the patient's body with the head. When adjusting the head, the patients chin is tucked to avoid skin folds on the back of the neck. The spine port should not exit through the mandible and oral cavity. Extended distance (SSD technique) is often used to achieve a greater field length for the spine

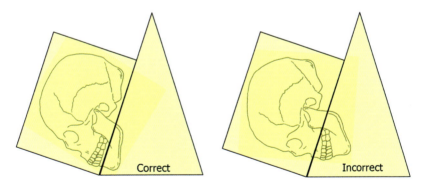

Correct   Incorrect

- The CNS is treated through two lateral head ports and a posterior spine port. When the entire length of the spine cannot be encompassed in a single port, it can be divided into two abutting ports. The collimator is rotated on the lateral head ports to match the divergence of the upper spine port

- When the two lateral head ports are setup, the table should be angled to match the upper spine port to the divergence of the lateral head ports

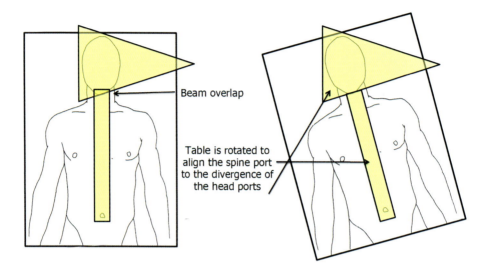

- To adequately encompass the posterior aspect of the retina and orbit while sparing the anterior portion of the globe and lens, a 4-5 degree gantry angle can be used to correct for divergence and create a straight line behind the eyes.

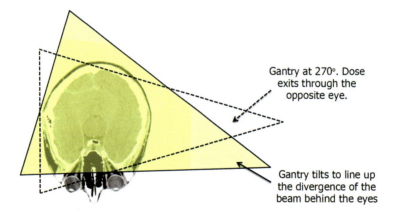

- To achieve the angle needed for this non-divergent beam behind the eyes, a BB can be placed on the outer canthus of one eye, and a wire can be placed on the outer canthus of the other eye. The gantry is rotated until the BB and the wire line up

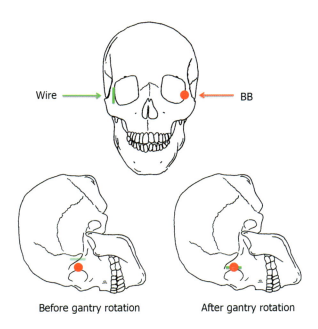

- Another technique for head ports is to position the isocenter on the canthi to minimize beam divergence (shielding the lenses)

- For table kicks and collimator angles, the appropriate number of degrees needed to turn can be determined using this formula:

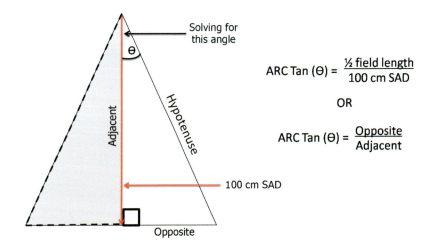

CNS Examples

A craniospinal irradiation technique consists of two lateral head ports and 2 posterior spine ports. The field dimensions are:

- Lateral head ports = 23 width x 22 length, treated at midline (8 cm depth, 100 SAD)

- The upper spine port is 7 cm x 20 cm, and the lower spine port is 14 cm x 24 cm to encompass the sacral nerves. These fields are treated at 100 SSD

Using the above information, solve for the following:

If the lateral head ports must be aligned to match the divergence of the upper spine port, how many degrees should the collimator be angled, and in what direction? (The collimator rotation for the brain field is determined by one-half the field length and the SSD of the upper spine port

$$\text{Collimator angle for brain field} = (\arctan) \frac{\tfrac{1}{2}\text{ upper spine length}}{100 \text{ SSD}}$$

$$\text{Collimator angle for brain field} = (\arctan) \frac{10}{100 \text{ SSD}}$$

$$\text{Collimator angle for brain field} = \boxed{11.3°}$$

The table angle needed for the PA spine to match the brain field is determined from the length of the brain port and where length is defined

$$\text{Table angle for PA spine} = (\arctan) \frac{\tfrac{1}{2}\text{ brain field length}}{100 \text{ SAD}}$$

$$\text{Table angle for PA spine} = (\arctan) \frac{11}{100 \text{ SAD}}$$

$$\text{Table angle} = \boxed{6.3°}$$

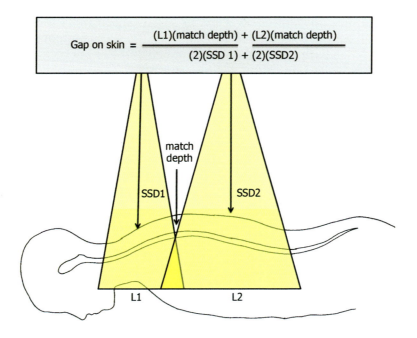

Gap Calculation Example

The upper spine port is 7 cm x 20 cm and the lower spine port is 14 cm x 24 cm to encompass the sacral nerves. Both fields are to be treated at 100 SSD. What is the skin gap if the two spine ports are matched at 5 cm below the skin?

$$\text{Gap on skin} = \frac{(L1)(\text{match depth})}{(2)(SSD\,1)} + \frac{(L2)(\text{match depth})}{(2)(SSD2)}$$

$$\text{Gap on skin} = \frac{(20)(5)}{(2)(100)} + \frac{(24)(5)}{(2)(100)}$$

$$\text{Gap on skin} = (10)(.05) + (12)(.05)$$

$$\text{Gap on skin} = \boxed{1.1 \text{ cm}}$$

- L1 = length of the first field (or width if this is the side to be matched, see next problem)
- L2 = length or width of the second field
- Match depth = depth beneath the surface where the fields meet
- SSD1 = distance from the source to where the first field is defined (SAD if isocentric, see next problem)
- SSD2 = distance from the source to where the second field is defined

A patient is treated with 2 abdominal ports side by side. One port was treated at 100 SSD to a depth of 11 cm using a 6 wide by 12 cm long field. The second treatment port is to be set up using a 10 cm wide by 15 cm long port at 100 SAD to a midline depth of 11 cm. What skin gap is required to assure that the ports match at a depth of 11 cm? (The ports are side by side therefore width must be used opposed to length)

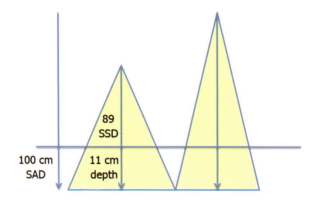

$$\text{Gap on skin} = \frac{(L1)(\text{match depth})}{(2)(SSD\ 1)} + \frac{(L2)(\text{match depth})}{(2)(SSD2)}$$

$$\text{Gap on skin} = \frac{(6)(11)}{(2)(100)} + \frac{(10)(11)}{(2)(100)}$$

$$\text{Gap on skin} = (3)(.11) + (5)(.11)$$

$$\text{Gap on skin} = \boxed{.88\ cm}$$

NOTE: This gap formula relies on the ratio of the field size to the source distance where the field is defined. The other variable required is depth at which the fields will match.

- The junction between the head and spine ports should be shifted 2-3 times during a course of treatment to avoid over or under dosage at the match. The fields are shifted by increasing or decreasing the field lengths without changing the central ray

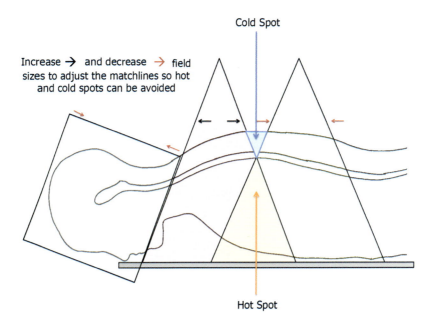

Brachytherapy

- The decay constant (λ) equals the total number of atoms that decay in a unit time. The relationship between the decay constant and the half life is:

    - $\lambda = 0.693 / t_{1/2}$

- Activity Calculations

    - Remaining activity (A) = Original Activity $(A_o)e^{-\lambda t}$

        - λ can also be substituted with $0.693/t_{1/2}$

        $$A = (A_o)e^{-(0.693/t_{1/2})(t)}$$

        - $t_{1/2}$ = half-life
        - t = time
        - A = new activity
        - A_o = original activity

Activity Example

A cesium 137 source received on September 30, 2010 had an activity of 61 mCi. What is the activity of the source 6 months later? ($t_{1/2}$ of Cs 137 = 30 years)

$$A = 61 \text{ mCi } (e^{(-.693/30 \text{ yrs})(0.5 \text{ yrs})})$$

$$A = 61 \text{ mCi } (.989)$$

$$A = \boxed{60.3 \text{ mCi}}$$

- Mean Life Calculations
    - Mean life calculations are used for brachytherapy sources with a short half life such as: I-125, Au–198, and Pd–103

    $$T = \frac{t_{1/2}}{\ln 2} = 1.442695 \, (t_{1/2})$$

    - where $1/\ln 2 = 1.442696$

Mean Life Example

110 mCi of Iodine-125 was implanted into the prostate. What is the radiation delivered or emitted? ($t_{1/2}$ of Iodine-125 = 59.4 days)

Mean life = 1.44 (59.4 days) = 85.5 days

Radiation delivered = 110 mCi (85.5 days) = $\boxed{9405 \text{ mCi}}$

- Exposure Rate Calculations
    - Applicable to a point source of radiation (distance of the source must be at least 5 times the length of the actual source)
    - Source length
        - Physical length - total length of source, including filtration
        - Active length - length of actual source, not including filtration

            Exposure rate = Gamma factor of isotope (Γ) x Activity x $(1/d^2)$

        - d = the distance from the source to the point of calculation

Exposure Rate Example

Calculate the exposure rate 11 cm away from an Iridium-192 source with an activity of 15 mCi. (Gamma factor of Ir-192 = 4.69 Roengten cm^2/mCi-hour)

Exposure rate = 4.69 Roengten cm^2/mCi-hr (15 mCi) (1/11^{2}cm) = .581 R/hr

.581 R/hr = 581 mR/hr

TD 5/5 Normal Tissue Tolerance Doses (Gy)
1.8-2.0 Gy/fraction (extracted from Emami, et.al., 1991 and National Cancer Institute publications)

Organ	1/3	2/3	3/3	End Point
Bladder	93	80	65	Symptomatic Contracture
Small Bowel	50	-	45	Obstruction/Perforation
Rectum	61	60	60	Proctitis/Necrosis/Stenosis/Fistula
Femoral Head and Neck	52	52	52	Necrosis
Large Bowel	55	-	45	Obstruction/Perforation/Ulceration/Fistula
Liver	50	35	30	Liver Failure
Kidney	50	35	23	Nephritis
Stomach	60	58	55	Ulceration/Perforation
Spinal Cord	50	50	47	Myelitis/Necrosis
Esophagus	60	58	55	Stricture/Perforation
Colon	55	-	45	Obstruction/Perforation/Ulceration/Fistula
Heart	60	45	40	Pericarditis
Lung	45	30	17	Pneumonitis
Thyroid	45	45	45	Thyroiditis
Larynx	45	45	45	Edema
Brachial Plexus	60	60	55	Nerve Damage
Lens of Eye	10	10	10	Cataract
Lacrimal Gland	26	26	26	Dry Eye
Optic Chiasm	50	50	50	Blindness
Optic Nerve	50	50	50	Blindness
Brain (Temporal Lobe)	58	51	47	Necrosis/Infarction
Brain Stem	60	53	50	Necrosis/Infarction
Ear	30/55	30/55	30/55	Acute/Chronic Serous Otitis
Parotid	32	32	32	Xerostomia
Temporomandibular Joint	61	60	60	Limitation of Joint Function

Practice Questions and Answers

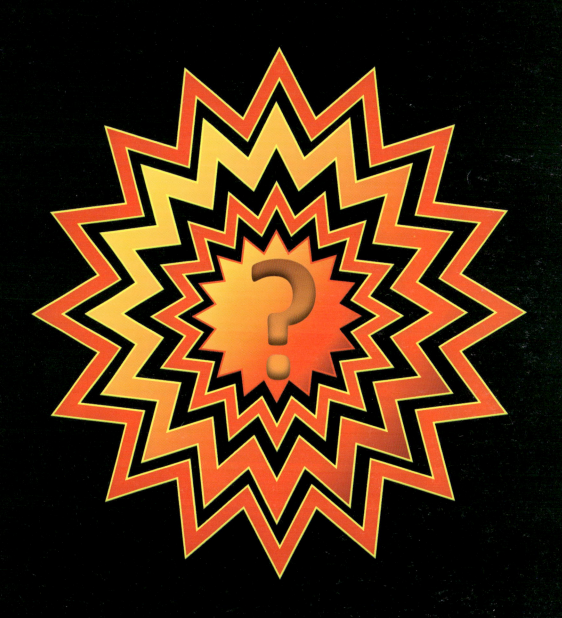

Practice Questions and Answers

1. Regarding linear accelerators, which of the following is TRUE?

    A. Maximum photon energy is equal to the energy of the electron striking the target
    B. The bending magnet is rotated out of the beam in the electron mode
    C. The beam current is higher in the electron mode than in the photon mode
    D. The scattering foil is the primary component for photon production → flattening Filter

2. 1 mSv is equal to _____ rem.

    A. 0.01
    B. 0.1
    C. 1.0
    D. 10

3. If the total body is exposed to a dose of 4500 cGy in a single exposure, the most likely cause of death would be:

    A. Infection and low blood counts
    B. Severe damage to the intestines
    C. Cerebral edema
    D. Death would not be likely with this dose

4. By what factor does the intensity decrease when someone moves from 10 meters to 20 meters away from a radioactive source?

    A. 2
    B. 4
    C. 10
    D. 20

5. What is the allowable cumulative exposure for a radiation worker?

    A. One rem times the worker's age in years
    B. Five rem times the worker's age in decades
    C. 100 rem times the worker's age in years
    D. Five rem times the worker's age in decades

6. Which of the following are interactions between an incident photon and an atomic nucleus?

    A. Photoelectric
    B. Compton
    C. Coherent
    D. Pair production

7. A barrier that attenuates the useful portion of the beam to the required degree is known as?

   A. Secondary Barrier
   B. Incident Shielding
   C. Tenth Value Layer
   D. Primary Barrier

8. A "star" shot on a linear accelerator is performed to test the rotational axis of the:
[1] collimator
[2] couch
[3] gantry

   A. 1 and 2 only
   B. 2 and 3 only
   C. 1 and 3 only
   D. 1, 2, and 3

9. Direct exposure to lasers that are used for patient alignment purposes can be a hazard for the:

   A. Pituitary
   B. Retina
   C. Commissure
   D. Inner Ear

10. The average photon beam energy produced by a 6 MV linear accelerator is approximately _____ MV:

   A. 2
   B. 4
   C. 6
   D. 9

11. Which of the following tissues arise from mesenchymal stem cells (MSC)?
[1] Blood
[2] Cartilage
[3] Bone

   A. 1 only
   B. 2 only
   C. 2 and 3 only
   D. 1, 2, and 3

12. In bremsstrahlung radiation, the incoming electron:

   A. interacts with an orbiting electron
   B. is deflected by the nucleus of the atom
   C. creates a positive and negative ion
   D. cascades to a lower energy state

13. Exposure is:

A. Measure of ionization in air
B. Known as a biological dose equivalent
C. The absorbed dose multiplied by the quality factor
D. The possibility of a random interaction

14. Which of the following does not ionize directly?

A. Proton
B. Neutron
C. Alpha particle
D. Electron

15. The half-life of cobalt-60 is:

A. 2.5 yrs
B. 3.2 yrs
C. 5.3 yrs
D. 8.2 yrs

16. Linear accelerators have which of the following type of target?

A. Hooded anode
B. Waveguide
C. Transmission
D. Rotating cathode

17. Klystrons and magnetrons are:

A. Radiation monitors
B. Microwave sources
C. Monitors used for mechanical motions
D. Beam shaping devices

18. Which the following is the most common metastatic site for prostate cancer?

A. Lung
B. Liver
C. Bone
D. Brain

19. The last part of the colon that leads into the rectum is known as the:

A. Ascending colon
B. Hepatic colon
C. Descending colon
D. Sigmoid colon

20. Why do high energy photon accelerators require flattening filters?

   A. To increase the penetrating ability of the beam
   B. To reduce dose rates to a safe level
   C. To filter out low energy photons
   D. To decrease the intensity along the central axis

21. Lead alone could be used in room shielding when the following interactions predominate:

   A. Photoelectric
   B. Bragg peak
   C. Pair production
   D. Compton scattering

22. The intensity of a radiation beam is measured at a distance of 100 cm and is found to be 150 cGy/min. What is the intensity of this beam at 105 cm?

   A. 136 cGy/min
   B. 143 cGy/min
   C. 157 cGy/min
   D. 165 cGy/min

23. What does ALARA mean?

   A. Acting responsibly as soon as required
   B. Advocating as little radiation as reasonably achievable
   C. Reporting all accidents as soon as discovered
   D. Always leaving an area right away

24. The most common thermoluminescence material used in radiation dosimetry is:

   A. $CaSO_4$
   B. LiF
   C. CaF_2
   D. Li_2B

25. The angle of the mandible is generally located at which cervical vertebra level?

   A. C-1
   B. C-3
   C. C-5
   D. C-7

26. The trachea is a hollow tube about 10 cm in length that extends from the larynx to a bifurcation called the:

A. Bronchus
B. Saphanous
C. Tributary
D. Carina

27. Monitoring of dose rate and field symmetry is best accomplished by using a (an):

A. Pocket dosimeter
B. Ion chamber
C. TLD
D. GM counter

28. In the pancreas, where do most tumors originate?

A. Head
B. Tail
C. Body
D. Hilum

29. Effects for which the severity of the effect in the individual varies with the radiation dose, and a threshold usually exists is called:

A. Stochastic - random
B. Deterministic
C. Acute
D. Protracted

30. Which of the following devices are used for area surveys:
[1] Ionization chambers
[2] Parallel-plate chambers
[3] Geiger-Mueller detectors

A. 1 and 2 only
B. 1 and 3 only
C. 2 and 3 only
D. 1, 2, and 3

31. According to NRC regulations, what is the MPD for those who are NOT trained radiation workers?

A. 0.1 rem/year
B. 1.0 rem/year
C. 1.25 rem/year
D. 5.0 rem/year

32. The categories of visitors who are excluded from visiting a radioactive iodine patient are:

   A. Females who have reproductive potential and children of any age
   B. Elderly females and children under 13 years of age
   C. No categories are excluded because radiation safety precautions are in effect
   D. Pregnant women and children under 18 years of age

33. The section of the bladder between the ureters and the urethra is known as the:

   A. Trigone
   B. Urogenital diaphragm
   C. Calyces
   D. Muscularis propria

34. Which is the largest paranasal sinus cavity?

   A. Nasopharynx
   B. Sphenoid
   C. Maxillary
   D. Frontal

35. Bolus can be used to:
[1] Flatten out surface irregularities
[2] Reduce beam penetration
[3] Increase surface dose

   A. 1 and 2 only
   B. 2 and 3 only
   C. 1 and 3 only
   D. 1, 2, and 3

36. According to AAPM TG-40, gantry/collimator angle indicators on the linear accelerator must agree within _____ degree(s).

   A. 1
   B. 2
   C. 3
   D. 5

37. Lung cancer frequently spreads to:
[1] Brain
[2] Pancreas
[3] Bone

   A. 1 and 2 only
   B. 2 and 3 only
   C. 1 and 3 only
   D. 1, 2, and 3

38. What is the purpose of the scattering foil in a linear accelerator?

A. Increase the intensity of the beam
B. Provide uniform electron fluence
C. Absorb radiation
D. Flatten out photon beam

39. What is the approximate Dmax of a 10 mV linear accelerator?

A. 1.0 cm
B. 1.5 cm   2.5
C. 2.0 cm
D. 2.5 cm

40. Photoelectric interactions of a 60 keV beam are greatest in:

A. Water → dependant on Z number
B. Fat
C. Muscle
D. Bone

41. Which of the following structures is most radiosensitive (susceptible to long term damage at the lowest dose)?

A. Spinal cord -47
B. Heart   40
C. Lung   17.5
D. Liver   30

42. The stomach is located in the:

A. Right upper quadrant
B. Right lower quadrant
C. Left upper quadrant
D. Left lower quadrant

43. What symptoms are most often associated with carcinoma of the cervix?
[1] Vaginal discharge
[2] Vaginal bleeding
[3] Bloating and weight gain

A. 1 and 2 only
B. 2 and 3 only
C. 1 and 3 only
D. 1, 2, and 3

-2

44. What does the oropharynx region include?
[1] Base of tongue
[2] Tonsil
[3] Soft palate

   A. 1 and 2 only
   B. 2 and 3 only
   C. 1 and 3 only
   D. 1, 2 and 3

45. From what type of tissue do most sarcomas arise?

   A. Epithelial
   B. Connective
   C. Nerve
   D. Skin

46. Referring to the MRI scan to the right, the outlined organ is/are the:

   A. Seminal vesicles
   B. Stomach
   C. Pancreas
   D. Spleen

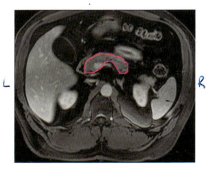

47. Where is a sarcoma most likely to metastasize?

   A. Bone
   B. Lung
   C. Blood
   D. Brain

48. When a patient presents with a bloody nasal discharge and a neck mass, the most likely diagnosis is:

   A. Larynx cancer
   B. Hypopharyngeal cancer
   C. Nasopharyngeal cancer
   D. Brain metastases

49. Which of the following is the most common primary brain tumor in adults?

   A. Glioma
   B. Meningioma
   C. Medulloblastoma
   D. Metastasis

50. With breast cancer which of the following patterns of lymph node drainage occurs most often?

   A. Internal mammary
   B. Axillary
   C. Supraclavicular
   D. Mediastinal

51. The most common site for metastatic spread of carcinoma of the penis is the:

   A. Inguinal nodes
   B. Periaortic nodes
   C. Lungs
   D. Liver

52. **Hypofractionation is:**
   [1] Treatment given in fewer fractions than standard
   [2] Use of very low dose rates
   [3] Treatment given two or more times per day

   A. 1 only
   B. 2 only
   C. 1 and 3 only
   D. 1, 2, and 3

53. **The epiglottis is a flap of cartilage that folds back to cover the entrance of the:**

   A. Hypopharynx
   B. Esophagus
   C. Trachea
   D. Larynx

54. **The most common histopathology of endometrial cancer is:**

   A. Adenocarcinoma
   B. Squamous cell
   C. Clear cell
   D. Mixed cellularity

55. **The largest lymphoid tissue is the:**

   A. Liver
   B. Spleen
   C. Thymus
   D. Jugulodiagastric node

56. In the normal adult male the prostate is located _____ to the bladder.

   A. Superior
   B. Inferior
   C. Posterior
   D. Anterior

57. Breast cancer metastasizes to:
[1] Bone
[2] Lung
[3] Brain

   A. 1 and 2 only
   B. 2 and 3 only
   C. 1 and 3 only
   D. 1, 2, and 3

58. The lower constricted portion of the uterus is called the:

   A. Endometrium
   B. Myometria
   C. Cervix
   D. Peritonial

59. The vocal cords are found within in a structure formed by cartilage called the:

   A. Pharynx
   B. Trachea
   C. Larynx
   D. Vallecula

60. What type of lung cancer may need prophylactic brain irradiation?

   A. Small cell
   B. Large cell
   C. Squamous cell
   D. Adenocarcinoma

61. What cancer is "peau de orange" associated with?

   A. Basal cell
   B. Melanoma
   C. Breast
   D. Prostate

62. The inguinal lymph nodes are generally included in which of the following treatment sites?

   A. Cervix
   B. Vulva
   C. Prostate
   D. Rectum

63. Nasopharyngeal tumors drain through what lymph node group first?

   A. Posterior cervical
   B. Submental
   C. Submaxillary
   D. Supraclavicular

64. The most common type of breast cancer is:

   A. Tubular
   B. Lobular
   C. Infiltrating ductal
   D. Adenoidcystic

65. Referring to the CT scan to the right, the arrow is pointing to the:

   A. Kidney
   B. Stomach
   C. Gallbladder
   D. Spleen

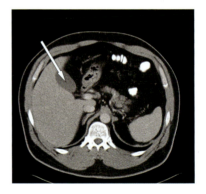

66. If a pathology report indicates a stage of T1N0M3, what can be said about the lymph node involvement of the nodes sampled?

   A. Positive nodes are found close to the primary tumor
   B. The nodes were unable to be sampled
   C. No positive nodes were present
   D. Positive nodes are found at distant sites

67. Which of the following is the most common site for a spinal cord compression?

   A. Cervical spine
   B. Thoracic spine
   C. Lumbar spine
   D. Sacrum

68. The tolerance dose (TD5/5) of the whole liver using standard fractionation (180-200 cGy/day) is:

   A. 1500-2000 cGy
   B. 2500-3000 cGy
   C. 3500-4000 cGy
   D. 4500-5000 cGy

69. The degree of cellular differentiation and rate of tumor growth is the:

   A. Stage
   B. Grade
   C. Etiology
   D. Epidemiology

70. When treating the entire CNS axis, the bottom of the spine port generally extends to the level of _____ when encompassing the cauda equina.

   A. L-3
   B. L-4
   C. L-5
   D. S-2

71. A multiple field technique (3 or more fields) is generally utilized when treating pituitary tumors, opposed to two lateral fields, to avoid an excessive dose to which of the following structures?

   A. Eyes
   B. Optic chiasm
   C. Temporal lobes
   D. Sella turcica

72. The common iliac nodes are generally found around the level of:

   A. C2
   B. T10
   C. L2
   D. L5

73. Where is the spleen located?

   A. Left upper quadrant (LUQ)
   B. Left lower quadrant (LLQ)
   C. Right upper quadrant (RUQ)
   D. Right lower quadrant (RLQ)

74. What external landmark can be used to localize the top of the larynx?

   A. Thyroid prominence
   B. Hyoid bone
   C. Cervical vertebrae
   D. Waldyer's ring

75. The collapse of a part or all of the lung, which often results from bronchial obstruction is termed:

   A. Bronchiectasis
   B. Atelectasis
   C. Pneumonitis
   D. Pleurisy

76. When treating the maxillary antrum, which neighboring structure is most sensitive?

   A. Eye
   B. Pituitary
   C. Spinal cord
   D. Brain

77. The pituitary is located:

   A. 2 cm posterior and 2 cm inferior to the external auditory meatus (EAM)
   B. 2 cm anterior and 2 cm superior to the EAM
   C. 1 cm posterior and 2 cm superior to the EAM
   D. 2 cm anterior and 2 cm inferior to the EAM

78. The trachea bifurcates at the level of:

   A. C4-C5
   B. T-12-L1
   C. T4-T5
   D. L4- L5

79. When treating a breast patient, the slope of the sternal notch to the xiphoid could be corrected by:

   A. Aquaplast
   B. Slant board
   C. Arm board
   D. Vaclok system

80. When treating a patient with cancer of the tongue, what is the purpose of putting a bite block (tongue gag) in the patient's mouth?

   A. Flatten tongue
   B. Protect teeth
   C. Localize mandible
   D. Alter dose distribution

81. What external landmark can be used to locate the carina?

   A. Thyroid prominence
   B. Axilla
   C. Angle of Louis
   D. Clavicle

82. The xiphoid is located at the level of:

    A. T4-T5
    B. T7-T8
    C. T9-T10
    D. T11-T12

83. The vallecula is located at the level of which of the following anatomical structures?

    A. Pyriform sinus
    B. Thyroid cartilage
    C. Hyoid bone
    D. Cricoid cartilage

84. The inferior border of a larynx port for a vocal cord carcinoma should anatomically correspond to:

    A. Bottom of thyroid cartilage
    B. Cricoid cartilage
    C. Hyoid bone
    D. First tracheal ring

85. If you are using a gonad shield when treating a patient with seminoma on a 6 MV linear accelerator, why can't all of the scatter to the testicles be eliminated?

    A. Internal scatter from the patient cannot be eliminated
    B. The shield would have to be too thick
    C. Part of the testicle must be exposed to properly treat the patient
    D. A 6 MV machine creates more scatter to the testicles when a testicular shield is used

86. What is the TD 5/5 tolerance dose using standard fractionation, for the lens of the eye?

    A. 450 cGy
    B. 1000 cGy
    C. 2000 cGy
    D. 5000 cGy

87. If a patient has a reaction to contrast media, you would expect to see all of the following EXCEPT:

    A. Hypotension
    B. Choking
    C. Incontinence
    D. Pruritis

88. The patient's chin is tilted down when treating a pituitary gland to avoid the:

   A. Eyes
   B. Surrounding brain tissue
   C. Spine
   D. Base of the skull

89. What is the technique in which a skin cancer is removed and examined one layer at a time?

   A. Curettage
   B. Cryosurgery
   C. Moh's surgery
   D. Dermobrasion

90. What type of lung cancer has the highest incidence of metastases at presentation?

   A. Small cell
   B. Large cell
   C. Squamous cell
   D. Adenocarcinoma

91. Which of the following areas are generally encompassed in a "German helmet" radiation port when treating acute lymphocytic leukemia?
[1] Cribiform plate
[2] Meninges
[3] Posterior retina

   A. 1 and 2 only
   B. 2 and 3 only
   C. 1 and 3 only
   D. 1, 2, and 3

92. A Strontium-90 applicator may be useful in the treatment of which of the following diseases of the eye?

   A. Retinoblastoma
   B. Malignant melanoma
   C. Pterygium
   D. Metastasis

93. The tolerance dose (TD 5/5) for the whole brain using standard fractionation is approximately:

   A. 3500 cGy
   B. 4500 cGy
   C. 5500 cGy
   D. 6500 cGy

94. Which of the following is the MOST radiosensitive structure?

   A. Liver
   B. Spine
   C. Brain stem
   D. Optic Chiasm

95. A non-osseous tumor of the bone marrow is:

   A. Fibrosarcoma
   B. Chonrosarcoma
   C. Osteosarcoma
   D. Multiple Myeloma

96. The false vocal cords are located _____ to the glottis.

   A. Anterior
   B. Posterior
   C. Superior
   D. Lateral

97. What is the primary reason to angle the gantry posteriorly when treating Grave's disease with two lateral fields?

   A. To avoid divergence into the lens
   B. To assure coverage of the posterior orbit
   C. To increase the dose to the orbital tissue
   D. To assure coverage of the protruding eye

98. What fraction would you multiply an electron energy by to estimate the 90% isodose range?

   A. 2/3
   B. 1/2
   C. 3/8
   D. 1/4

99. A patient is to receive 300 cGy per day on a Cobalt-60 unit through a single posterior field. The dose rate in air at 80 cm is 105.3 cGy/min and the backscatter factor is 1.029. The percent depth dose is 87.5%. Find the treatment time to deliver the prescribed dose.

   A. 4 min 22 sec
   B. 3 min 12 sec
   C. 3 min 10 sec
   D. 2 min 34 sec

100. A patient is usually treated at 100 cm SSD. The patient must be treated on a stretcher at 135 SSD. For the tumor dose and size treatment area to remain the same as originally planned, which of the following statements is true?
[1] The collimator setting will decrease
[2] The monitor unit setting will increase
[3] The exit dose will slightly increase

    A. 1 and 2 only
    B. 2 and 3 only
    C. 1 and 3 only
    D. 1, 2, and 3

101. A dose of 200 cGy is to be delivered at a depth of 10 cm at 100 SAD, from a single 15x15 cm field with 6 mV x-rays. Given the information below, what would the treatment monitor units be?

TMR (15x15 cm., depth 10 cm) = 0.806
Output in air, 100 SAD, 15x15 cm field size = 1.015 cGy/mu
BSF (15x15 cm) = 1.044
PDD (100 SSD, 15x15 cm, depth = 10 cm) = 72.2%

    A. 234 mu
    B. 245 mu
    C. 251 mu
    D. 273 mu

102. The depth of maximum dose is most dependent on:

    A. SSD
    B. Field size
    C. Beam energy
    D. Thickness of tissue

103. A 3.5 cm block on a blocking tray 45 cm from the source will block what width at 100 cm?

    A. 4.80 cm
    B. 5.20 cm
    C. 6.01 cm
    D. 7.78 cm

104. Why is a tumor of the parotid gland frequently treated with a ipsilateral beam arrangement?

    A. To avoid the spine
    B. To avoid the eyes
    C. To avoid the other parotid
    D. For ease of setup

105. What is the therapeutic ratio if the normal tissue tolerance is 5000 cGy and the lethal dose for the tumor is 4000?

   A. 0.80
   B. 1.25
   C. 1.56
   D. 2.10

106. Backscatter factors are independent of:

   A. Field size
   B. Radiation quality
   C. SSD
   D. TAR at dmax

107. A patient was mistakenly treated at 90 cm SSD instead of 100 cm due to a misaligned ODI. The prescribed dose was 2.5 Gy. What did the patient actually receive?

   A. 2.03 Gy
   B. 2.77 Gy
   C. 3.09 Gy
   D. 3.76 Gy

108. Areas outside the target that receives a higher dose than the specified target dose are called:

   A. Max target area
   B. Irradiated volume
   C. Hot spots
   D. Treated volume

109. A treatment time of 2.0 minutes requires that you add a wedge with a factor of 0.5, what will be the new treatment time?

   A. 1.0 min.
   B. 2.0 min.
   C. 2.5 min.
   D. 4.0 min.

110. Find the equivalent square of the resultant field of an 12 x 12 field with a 4 x 6 block.

   A. 8.0 x 8.0
   B. 9.0 x 9.0
   C. 10.0 x 10.0
   D. 11.0 x 11.0

111. A patient is 20 cm thick. You are to give 3000 cGy to midline weighted 2:1/right to left. The %dd for a depth of 10 cm is .641. What is the given dose to the left side?

   A. 1560 cGy
   B. 2340 cGy
   C. 3120 cGy
   D. 4680 cGy

112. A treatment of 137 monitor units requires that a blocking tray factor of 0.963 be included in the calculation. What are the correct treatment monitor units if the tray is added?

   A. 132 mu
   B. 137 mu
   C. 142 mu
   D. 150 mu

113. If a patient received a tumor dose of 250 cGy per day at the 79.2% dd, what is the daily maximum subcutaneous dose?

   A 198 cGy
   B. 250 cGy
   C. 316 cGy
   D. 405 cGy

114. A patient's prescription requires a total of 180 cGy to be delivered per day to equally weighted POP fields. The treatment time to deliver 100 cGy is 2.15 minutes. What treatment time must be delivered to each field to follow the prescription?

   A. 0.87 min.
   B. 1.94 min.
   C. 2.15 min.
   D. 3.88 min.

115. What precautions should be taken when treating the chest of a patient with a pacemaker?
[1] Cover the region of the pacemaker with lead
[2] Keep the pacemaker out of the direct beam, if possible
[3] Contact the manufacturer regarding radiation tolerance

   A. 1 and 2 only
   B. 2 and 3 only
   C. 1 and 3 only
   D. 1, 2 and 3

116. The largest salivary gland in the head and neck is the:

   A. Submaxillary
   B. Sublinguinal
   C. Parotid
   D. Mastoid

117. When performing a CT on a patient for IMRT treatment of a prostate, what size slices are used through the true pelvis?

   A. 5.0 mm
   B. 3.0 mm
   C. 1.0 mm
   D. 10 mm

118. The practical range for 18 MeV electrons is:

   A. 6 cm
   B. 8 cm
   C. 9 cm
   D. unable to determine

119. When treating with orthovoltage X-rays, the percentage depth dose will increase with all of the following EXCEPT:

   A. Increasing the field size
   B. Increasing the kV
   C. Increasing the mA
   D. Increasing the distance

120. A patient is accidentally treated at 78 cm SSD, instead of 80 cm SSD. The treatment depth is 3 cm. If the prescribed tumor dose is 200 cGy through a single field, what dose did the tumor actually receive?

   A. 190 cGy
   B. 195 cGy
   C. 205 cGy
   D. 210 cGy

121. The most common presentation of superior vena cava syndrome is:

   A. Distended veins in the head and neck
   B. Bloody nasal discharge
   C. Headaches
   D. Incontinence

122. For patients with bladder cancer, the bladder should be _____ during treatment, when the entire bladder is the target volume.

　A. Empty
　B. Partially full
　C. Full
　D. Localized with contrast media

123. The rapid fall off of dose around a cesium-137 source in a 5cm radius of tissue is due primarily to:
[1] The inverse square law
[2] The low energy of the radiation
[3] Alpha and beta emission

　A. 1 only
　B. 2 only
　C. 3 only
　D. 1, 2, and 3

124. When manipulating a CT image, increasing the width of the window:
[1] Decreases contrast
[2] Increases latitude
[3] Increases speed

　A. 1 and 2 only
　B. 2 and 3 only
　C. 1 and 3 only
　D. 1, 2 and 3

125. What would be the TD 5/5 tolerance dose for both whole lungs given in fractions of 180 cGy/day?

　A. 1500-2500 cGy
　B. 2500-3500 cGy
　C. 3500-4500 cGy
　D. 4500-5000 cGy

126. The amount of energy transferred to a material per unit length of travel is termed:

　A. RBE
　B. LET
　C. QF
　D. OER

127. What is the TD 5/5 tolerance dose for the whole kidney given in fractions of 180 cGy/day?

　A. 1500-2000 cGy
　B. 2000-2500 cGy
　C. 2500-3000 cGy
　D. 3000-3500 cGy

128. What is the dose at which you generally reduce the field "off cord" when treating a head and neck cancer?

    A. 3000-3500 cGy
    B. 4500-5000 cGy
    C. 5500-6000 cGy
    D. 6000-6500 cGy

129. RBE is dependent on which of the following:
[1] Radiation quality
[2] Radiation dose per fraction
[3] Tissue irradiated

    A. 1 and 2 only
    B. 2 and 3 only
    C. 1 and 3 only
    D. 1, 2 and 3

130. When dealing with OER and anoxic tissue, which would be the most effective?

    A. 6 mV photons
    B. Protons
    C. Neutrons
    D. Electrons

131. What normal organ would be at most risk when treating a maxillary sinus tumor?

    A. Oral cavity
    B. Pituitary gland
    C. Eye
    D. Ear

132. A patient is setup on a wing board with both arms up. What areas are commonly treated using this position?
[1] Breast
[2] Lung
[3] Pancreas

    A. 1 and 2 only
    B. 2 and 3 only
    C. 1 and 3 only
    D. 1, 2 and 3

133. What is the most potent chemical modifier of radiosensitivity to X and gamma rays?

    A. 5FU
    B. Oxygen
    C. Misonidazole
    D. Adriamycin

134. A patient was treated with a 20 cm long field and a 15 cm long field is matched to it. Both fields are set at 80 SSD. What is the gap on the skin if the fields are to be matched at 10 cm depth?

   A. 0.9 cm
   B. 1.3 cm
   C. 1.8 cm
   D. 2.2 cm

135. When a patient has been treated with a cesium insertion for cervical cancer, why would she be treated with external beam radiation following the cesium?

   A. To decrease the size of the tumor
   B. To deliver a higher dose to the cervix
   C. To avoid infertility
   D. To treat the pelvic lymph nodes

136. A patient is treated with a 8x15 cm field, Co-60 unit, 80 cm SSD to a depth of 5 cm, 78.5% dd. What would the percentage depth dose be if the SSD was changed to 100 cm?

   A. 76.9%
   B. 80.1%
   C. 90.2%
   D. 96.1%

137. A patient thickness is measured to be 20 cm anterior to posterior. If the patient is brought to an SSD of 90 cm on a 100 cm SAD accelerator, what should a ruler read from the tabletop to isocenter? Assume the patient is flat on the table.

   A. 10 cm
   B. 15 cm
   C. 20 cm
   D. Cannot determine from information

138. Which of the following is required for fabricating custom cut blocks?
[1] Source axis distance
[2] Source image distance
[3] Source to block tray distance

   A. 1 and 2 only
   B. 2 and 3 only
   C. 1 and 3 only
   D. 1, 2 and 3

139. The collimators on a linear accelerator are calibrated for a distance of 100 cm. To obtain a field size of 30 cm x 30 cm at 80 cm, what collimator setting is required?

   A. 26.7 cm x 26.7 cm
   B. 30.0 cm x 30.0 cm
   C. 37.5 cm x 37.5 cm
   D. 41.0 cm x 41.0 cm

140. When treating a lesion on the outside of the nose with electrons, what is the major reason that you place a wax-coated lead strip in the nose?

   A. To increase the dose on the outside of the nose
   B. To decrease the dose to the inside of the nose
   C. For patient comfort
   D. A lead strip should never be placed within the nose

141. A dose of 3000 cGy is delivered to a depth of 8 cm at PDD of 76%. What is the dose to an underlying organ at 14 cm at a PDD of 58%?

   A. 5172 cGy
   B. 2289 cGy
   C. 3947 cGy
   D. 4231 cGy

142. Assume a half value layer of Pb = 3 mm. How thick would the lead have to be to reduce exposure of 100 mR at 4 meters to 100 mR at one meter?

   A. 12 mm
   B. 9 mm
   C. 6 mm
   D. 3 mm

143. A patient is to be treated isocentrically to his midline on the 6 MV linear accelerator at 100 cm SAD. Calipers have measured the patient thickness to be 21 cm. The patient is positioned flat on the table top. What SSD is required for isocentric treatment to the patient's midline?

   A. 79 cm
   B. 89.5 cm
   C. 100 cm
   D. 110.5 cm

144. The output of a Cobalt-60 teletherapy unit is 85 cGy/min in air at 80.5 cm for an 11 x 11 field. The backscatter factor for this field is 1.10. Calculate the time necessary to deliver a dose of 170 cGy at a depth of 8 cm, 80 SSD. The PDD for an 11 x 11 field at a depth of 8 cm is 63%.

   A. 2.06 min
   B. 2.53 min
   C. 2.89 min
   D. 3.46 min

145. Two wedges are used to treat a maxillary antrum tumor through an anterior and a lateral port. What part of the wedges should be adjacent?

A. Thin side anterior to thick side laterally
B. Thin side anterior to thin side laterally
C. Thick side anterior to thick side laterally
D. Thick side anterior to thin side laterally

146. When treating the breast, if a slant board is used rather than the patient lying flat, which of the following is TRUE?

A. The breast "falls" into the supraclavicular port
B. More lung tissue is included in the supraclavicular port
C. It is more difficult for the patient to raise her arm
D. The chest wall cannot be treated when the slant board is used

147. To verify that the radiation field and the light field are aligned on a 10 MV linear accelerator you could use the following:

A. Tissue equivalent phantom and an ionization chamber
B. Mechanical distance indicator and paper
C. A shielding block and readi-pak x-ray film
D. Readi-pak x-ray film, a pen and a ruler

148. Calculate the monitor units to deliver 200 cGy to the 90% isodose line using 12 MeV electrons at 100 SSD if the measured output for the cone and cutout is .787 cGy/MU at 100 SSD.

A. 255 MU
B. 229 MU
C. 282 MU
D. 301 MU

149. A patient is receiving 300 cGy per day to a spinal cord lesion at 89.5 percent depth dose. What is the daily given dose at dmax?

A. 269
B. 335
C. 400
D. not enough information to calculate

150. For photon energies between 0.150 MeV and 10.0 MeV, the predominant type of interaction is:

A. Photoelectric
B. Compton
C. Pair Production
D. Bremsstrahlung

151. All of the following data was obtained using a 15x15 cm field size at 100 SAD. The dose at dmax in tissue is 280 cGy. The BSF is 1.031 and the TMR at a depth of 12 cm is .721. Find the dose delivered at 12 cm depth through a single 15x15 cm field at 100 SAD.

   A. 388 cGy
   B. 208 cGy
   C. 202 cGy
   D. 196 cGy

152. Which of the following systems must be functioning in order to treat a patient safely on a high energy machine?
[1] A two-way audio system
[2] A visual system to monitor the patient and machine function
[3] An audible signal to inform the patient when the machine is on

   A. 1 and 2 only
   B. 1 and 3 only
   C. 2 and 3 only
   D. 1, 2 and 3

153. To preserve the skin sparing properties of the megavoltage photon beams, the compensator is placed at least _____ from the skin.

   A. 1-5 cm
   B. 5-10 cm
   C. 9-12 cm
   D. 15-20 cm

154. The PDD for a 12 x 12 cm field, 6 MV, 5 cm depth at 80 cm SSD is 82.8%. Calculate the percent depth dose for the same field size and depth for 100 cm SSD.

   A. 81.4%
   B. 82.1%
   C. 83.4 %
   D. 84.2 %

155. What is the main advantage of using Cerrobend over lead in custom blocking?

   A. It is softer than lead
   B. It cannot form air bubbles
   C. It has a lower melting point
   D. It requires thicker blocks to obtain the same effect

156. Portal verification is defined as the documentation of :

   A. Isodose curves through the use of film or electronic imaging devices
   B. The extent of disease using film or electronic imaging devices
   C. The actual treatment using film or electronic imaging devices
   D. The approval of the treatment port by a qualified physician

157. The patient is positioned supine and is to be treated using an isocentric technique. The AP SSD reads 88 cm and you move the isocenter 2 cm posteriorly. What should the SSD read?

A. 86 cm
B. 88 cm
C. 90 cm
D. Unable to determine

158. The patient is positioned supine and is to be treated using an isocentric technique. The AP SSD reads 84 cm. If the patient's thickness is 36 cm, what is the PA SSD?

A. 64 cm
B. 80 cm
C. 84 cm
D. 88 cm

159. According to the ICRU terminology, the area that is defined as the palpable or visible extent of the malignant tumor is called the:

A. Treated volume
B. Gross tumor volume
C. Clinical target volume
D. Planning target volume

160. What is the tolerance dose for the outlined organ in the MRI to the right?

A. 2500-3000 cGy
B. 3000-3500 cGy
C. 4500-5000 cGy
D. 6000-6500 cGy

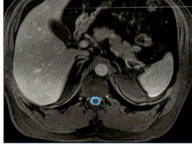

161. Calculate the dose at dmax if 200 cGy is delivered to 7 cm below the skin at the 72 percent depth dose.

A. 144 cGy
B. 197 cGy
C. 206 cGy
D. 278 cGy

162. A lung lesion is being treated using POP isocentric ports with the patient in the supine position. The physician wants to place the isocenter at the patient's midline. The ruler placed on the table top reads 30 cm from the table top to the patient's anterior surface. There is a 1.5 cm immobilization device between the patient and the table. What is the patient's total thickness?

   A. 30 cm
   B. 28.5 cm
   C. 14.3 cm
   D. Unable to determine

163. The collimator setting is 8 cm x 10 cm on a 100 cm SAD machine. The SSD on the patient's skin reads 90 cm. What is the field size on the patient's skin?

   A. 7.2 cm x 9.0 cm
   B. 8.0 cm x 10.0 cm
   C. 8.9 cm x 11.1 cm
   D. Unable to determine

164. You have an extremely large patient and you must treat two lateral pelvic fields. What technique will give you the most even dose distribution throughout the treatment field?

   A. Isocentric technique treated to the patient's midline
   B. SSD technique, moving the treatment table as far away from the source as possible
   C. Midline isocentric technique with blocks added
   D. Midline isocentric technique with wedges added

165. A patient is treated on the 6 MV linear accelerator. The patient is setup to 94 cm SSD. The TAR at 6 cm depth is 0.87 and the output at isocenter in air is 1.02 cGy/MU for the required field size. How many monitor units will it take to deliver 100 cGy to a depth of 6 cm?

   A. 88 MU
   B. 102 MU
   C. 113 MU
   D. 116 MU

166. A treatment designed to be given at 100 SSD is mistakenly given at 94 SSD. What is the error in dose delivered?

   A. 13% overdose
   B. 13% underdose
   C. 6% overdose
   D. 6% underdose

167. When a field size is changed during the course of a patient's treatment, which of the following statements are TRUE?
[1] Treatment depth must change
[2] The physician must include changes in the prescription
[3] The monitor units or time must be recalculated

    A. 1 and 2 only
    B. 1 and 3 only
    C. 2 and 3 only
    D. 1, 2 and 3

168. All chemicals used in a department require:

    A. Listing with the human resource department
    B. Material safety data sheets (MSDS)
    C. An 800 number for toxic information
    D. Labels containing information in case of exposure

169. The standard amount of time that should elapse between two radiation therapy treatments given in the same day to the same site is:

    A. 3 hours
    B. 6 hours
    C. 9 hours
    D. 12 hours

170. If 1.5 cm is added to the inferior border of a treatment port, what happens to the original isocenter if you are not using independent (asymmetric) jaws?

    A. Shifts 0.75 cm superiorly
    B. Shifts 0.75 cm inferiorly
    C. Shifts 1.5 cm superiorly
    D. Isocenter stays the same

171. Which of the following statements concerning patient's rights are TRUE?
[1] A relative has the right to access a patient's record
[2] The patient has the right to refuse treatment
[3] The patient has the right to be informed of any alternative procedures prior to his treatment

    A. 1 and 2 only
    B. 2 and 3 only
    C. 1 and 3 only
    D. 1, 2 and 3

172. MV portal films taken on a megavoltage machine have less contrast than kV films because the MV image results principally from:

A. Pair production
B. Photoelectric effect
C. Compton interaction
D. Photodisintegration

173. Restraining a patient in an aquaplast mask without consent can be considered:
[1] Battery
[2] Assault
[3] Humane

A. 1 and 2 only
B. 2 and 3 only
C. 3 only
D. 1, 2 and 3

174. During radiation therapy to the pelvis if a patient is complaining of the following, which would most likely warrant interruption in the course of treatment:

A. Dysuria
B. Acute radiation enteritis
C. Tenesmus
D. Impotence

175. Which of the following is TRUE concerning a patient's medical record?
[1] It is a legal public document
[2] Patient's may review their record upon request
[3] It may be subpoenaed into a court of law

A. 1 and 2 only
B. 2 and 3 only
C. 1 and 3 only
D. 1, 2 and 3

176. The deficiency in the number of circulating white blood cells in the body is called:

A. Anemia
B. Leukopenia
C. Polycythemia
D. Thrombcytopenia

177. After what time period would fibrosis generally appear following standard external beam therapy?

A. One month
B. One year
C. One week
D. Two weeks

178. When treating the parotid gland with standard fractionation (180-200 cGy/day), what is the tolerance dose (TD 5/5) that patients will develop xerostomia?

A. 500-1500 cGy
B. 2500-3500 cGy
C. 4500-5500 cGy
D. 6500-7500 cGy

179. The most common long term effect of radiation therapy to the lung is:

A. Pneumonitis
B. Necrosis
C. Fibrosis
D. Esophagitis

180. When treating a patient with glioblastoma, he begins to experience nausea, dizziness, and blurred vision. Which is the most likely reason?

A. Tumor necrosis
B. Cerebral edema
C. CNS syndrome
D. Reaction to medication

181. Deodorants should not be used on the skin within a radiation treatment field because the deodorants will:

A. Create scatter radiation
B. Act as a bolus
C. Enhance the radiation
D. Irritate sensitive skin

182. Written defamation of character is best known as:

A. Slander
B. Libel
C. Cursing
D. Literary fault

183. The normal platelet count is approximately:

A. 60,000 cc
B. 80,000 cc
C. 120,000 cc
D. 300,000 cc

184. All of the following medications are antiemetics except:

A. Norazine
B. Compazine
C. Tylenol
D. Torecan

185. Bone marrow depression is most likely to occur when you are treating which part of the body?

A. Skull
B. Pelvic bones
C. Femur
D. Vertebrae

186. Which of the following chemotherapeutic drugs sensitizes the human heart?

A. Bleomycin
B. Adriamycin
C. Vincristine
D. Cis-platinum

187. When treating the whole brain which drug is used to reduce radiation induced edema?

A. Antibiotics
B. Corticosteroids
C. Diuretics
D. Antihistamines

188. Patients who are neutropenic frequently present with _____ due to this condition:

A. Headaches
B. Shortness of breath
C. Bleeding
D. Infections

189. Which of the following types of medical apparatus should normally remain at a level above the patient at all times?

A. Chest tubes
B. Suction apparatus
C. Intravenous infusion equipment
D. Urinary drainage equipment

190. Which of the following is not a principle of using proper body mechanics?

A. Roll or slide objects when possible rather than lift
B. Keep the feet close together to provide support
C. Avoid twisting or bending at the waist
D. Lift objects with knees flexed

191. Which of the following methods is used to deliver hyperalimentation?

A. Oral intake
B. Intramuscular injection
C. Intravenous injection
D. Subcutaneous injection

192. The purpose of Protective (Reverse) Isolation is:

A. To prevent the transmission of pathogens in the feces
B. To prevent transmission of pathogens transmitted by direct contact with wounds
C. To protect an uninfected patient with lowered resistance
D. To prevent infection of personnel

193. Which of the following is the best method to prevent the spread of infection?

A. Wash hands
B. Wear gowns
C. Wear a mask
D. Clean the table

194. To prevent the spread of airborne droplet infection, which of the following must be employed?
[1] Gowns
[2] Masks
[3] Gloves

A. 1 only
B. 2 only
C. 3 only
D. 1, 2, and 3

195. The term that best describes the complete removal of all microorganisms is called:

   A. Medical asepsis
   B. Disinfection
   C. Antisepsis
   D. Sterilization

196. A patient with tuberculosis should be placed in:

   A. Enteric isolation
   B. Protective isolation
   C. Respiratory isolation
   D. Reverse isolation

197. Regarding "flatness" of a megavoltage photon beam, which of the following is TRUE?
[1] Beam flatness changes with depth due to scatter and decreased intensity at the field edge
[2] Adequate flatness is defined as +/- 3% over 80% of the field at the measured depth
[3] Flatness profiles may be used to determine symmetry

   A. 1 and 2 only
   B. 2 and 3 only
   C. 1 and 3 only
   D. 1, 2, and 3

198. During a convulsive seizure, the most important action to be taken by a therapist is:

   A. Prevent patient injury
   B. Give the patient water
   C. Give the patient sugar
   D. Hold the patient's tongue

199. A patient's separation is 30 cm. If the posterior SSD reads 89 cm on a 100 cm isocentric machine, what should the anterior SSD read?

   A. 70 cm
   B. 81 cm
   C. 89 cm
   D. unable to determine

200. An iatrogenic infection is one caused by:

   A. Hospital employees
   B. Synergistic effect with radiation
   C. Blood borne pathogens
   D. Complications from treatment

201. The point of intersection of the collimators and the gantry axis of rotation is the:

A. Midline
B. Isocenter
C. Treatment volume
D. Tumor volume

202. The two major energies associated with Cobalt -60 beta decay are gamma energies of:

A. 1.02 and 1.11 MeV
B. 1.17 and 1.33 MeV
C. 2.25 and 2.38 MeV
D. 2.51 and 3.02 MeV

203. The 80% isodose line can be estimated for electrons by dividing the energy (E) by:

A. 2.11
B. 2.33
C. 3.00
D. 4.00

204. According to the definition of the International Commission on Radiation Units and Measurements (ICRU), the wedge angle refers to: "the angle through which an isodose curve is titled at the central ray of a beam at a specified depth." The recommended depth is:

A. 5 cm
B. 10 cm
C. 15 cm
D. 20 cm

205. If you compare the penumbra of a 6 MV linear accelerator, operating in the photon mode, to the penumbra of a Co60 teletherapy machine using the same SSD, which of the following is TRUE?

A. The 6 MV linear accelerator has a greater penumbra than the Co-60 source
B. The 6 MV linear accelerator has less penumbra than the Co-60 source
C. The 6 MV linear accelerator has the same amount of penumbra as the Co-60
D. Neither machine would have measurable penumbra

206. Percentage depth dose increases with:
[1] Field size
[2] SSD
[3] Energy

A. 1 and 2 only
B. 2 and 3 only
C. 1 and 3 only
D. 1, 2, and 3

207. For radiation workers, the occupational dose is usually reported in:

　　A. Rad
　　B. Rem
　　C. Roentgen
　　D. Gray

208. A localization film was taken at 109 cm FFD. A 3.5 cm magnification ring was placed on the patient's skin. It measures 4.2 cm on the film. What distance is the magnification ring from the focal spot?

　　A. 83.2 cm
　　B. 90.8 cm
　　C. 138 cm
　　D. 147 cm

209. When a patient is treated with more than one beam, misalignment between parallel opposed beams can occur due to displacement of the:
[1] Target
[2] Collimator axis of rotation
[3] Gantry axis of rotation

　　A. 1 and 2 only
　　B. 2 and 1 only
　　C. 1 and 3 only
　　D. 1, 2, and 3

210. Which of the following has the LEAST radiosensitivity (most resistant)?

　　A. Bone marrow
　　B. Lymphoid tissue
　　C. Muscle
　　D. Mature cartilage

211. Where are pancoast tumors located?

　　A. Apex of lung
　　B. Periphery of lung
　　C. Mediastinum
　　D. Hilum

212. The most radiosensitive stage of the cell cycle is:

　　A. DNA synthesis
　　B. G1
　　C. G2
　　D. Mitosis

213. A split beam technique in which half of the field is blocked:
[1] Prevents beam divergence
[2] Allows for fields to match at the central ray
[3] Overlays the penumbra of two fields

   A. 1 and 2 only
   B. 1 and 3 only
   C. 2 and 3 only
   D. 1,2, and 3

214. The most common presenting sign of Wilms tumor is:

   A. Fever and chills
   B. Non-tender mass
   C. Bone pain
   D. Nausea and vomiting

215. In general, when treating with radiation, the proximal and distal margin around a soft tissue sarcoma should be at least _____ cm.

   A. 2
   B. 5
   C. 8
   D. 12

216. Where does the spinal cord start and stop in normal adults?

   A. Foramen magnum to L-5
   B. C-7 to L-5
   C. Foramen magnum to L-2
   D. Foramen magnum to T-12

217. The practical range of an electron beam :
[1] Increases with increasing electron energy
[2] About 1 cm for every 2 MEV
[3] About one half of the electron energy

   A. 1 and 2 only
   B. 2 and 3 only
   C. 1 and 3 only
   D. 1, 2, and 3

218. Mayneord's F factor is a correction for which of the following:

   A. Depth
   B. Field size
   C. Beam energy
   D. Distance

219. In a 120 degree arc rotation technique, the center of the high dose zone would be:

A. Deeper than the isocenter
B. Displaced towards the surface
C. Same shape as a 360 degree rotation
D. At the isocenter

220. Regarding electron beams which of the following is TRUE:
[1] Directly ionizing due to their negative charge
[2] Less likely to interact with air than photons
[3] Have a higher LET than photons

A. 1 and 2 only
B. 2 and 3 only
C. 1 and 3 only
D. 1, 2, and 3

1. A	39. D	77. B
2. B	40. D	78. C
3. C	41. C	79. B
4. B	42. C	80. A
5. A	43. A	81. C
6. D	44. D	82. C
7. D	45. B	83. C
8. D	46. C	84. B
9. B	47. B	85. A
10. A	48. C	86. B
11. D	49. A	87. C
12. B	50. B	88. A
13. A	51. A	89. C
14. B	52. A	90. A
15. C	53. D	91. D
16. C	54. A	92. C
17. B	55. B	93. B
18. C	56. B	94. A
19. D	57. D	95. D
20. D	58. C	96. C
21. A	59. C	97. A
22. A	60. A	98. D
23. B	61. C	99. C
24. B	62. B	100. D
25. B	63. A	101. A
26. D	64. C	102. C
27. B	65. C	103. D
28. A	66. C	104. C
29. B	67. B	105. B
30. B	68. B	106. C
31. A	69. B	107. C
32. D	70. D	108. C
33. A	71. C	109. D
34. C	72. D	110. D
35. D	73. A	111. A
36. A	74. A	112. C
37. C	75. B	113. C
38. B	76. A	114. B

115. D	153. D	191. C
116. C	154. D	192. C
117. B	155. C	193. A
118. C	156. C	194. B
119. C	157. A	195. D
120. D	158. B	196. C
121. A	159. B	197. D
122. A	160. C	198. A
123. A	161. D	199. B
124. A	162. B	200. D
125. A	163. A	201. B
126. B	164. B	202. B
127. B	165. C	203. C
128. B	166. A	204. B
129. D	167. C	205. B
130. B	168. B	206. D
131. C	169. B	207. B
132. D	170. B	208. B
133. B	171. B	209. D
134. D	172. C	210. D
135. D	173. A	211. A
136. B	174. B	212. D
137. A	175. D	213. A
138. B	176. B	214. B
139. C	177. B	215. B
140. B	178. B	216. C
141. B	179. C	217. D
142. A	180. B	218. D
143. B	181. D	219. B
144. C	182. B	220. C
145. C	183. D	
146. B	184. C	
147. D	185. B	
148. C	186. B	
149. B	187. B	
150. B	188. D	
151. C	189. C	
152. A	190. B	

Notes